Practical Emergency Ophthalmology Handbook

An Algorithm Based Approach to Ophthalmic Emergencies

T0186348

Practical Emergency Ophthalmology Handbook

An Algorithm Based Approach to Ophthalmic Emergencies

Edited by
Dr. Amy-lee Shirodkar
Dr. Gwyn Samuel Williams

illustrated by Bushra Thajudeen

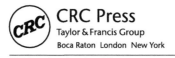

CRC Press
Taylor & Francis Group
Boca Raton London New York

CRC Press is an imprint of the
Taylor & Francis Group, an **informa** business

CRC Press
Taylor & Francis Group
6000 Broken Sound Parkway NW, Suite 300
Boca Raton, FL 33487-2742

© 2020 by Taylor & Francis Group, LLC
CRC Press is an imprint of Taylor & Francis Group, an Informa business

No claim to original U.S. Government works

Printed on acid-free paper

International Standard Book Number-13: 978-0-367-11027-7 (Paperback)
978-0-367-13503-4 (Hardback)

Library of Congress Cataloging-in-Publication Data

Names: Shirodkar, Amy-lee, editor. | Williams, Gwyn (Ophthalmologist), editor.
Title: Practical emergency ophthalmology handbook / edited by Dr. Amy-lee Shirodkar, Dr. Gwyn Samuel Williams.
Description: Boca Raton : CRC Press, [2020] | Includes bibliographical references and index. | Summary: "This handbook is designed to help clinician or trainee and guide them toward the right decision-making pathway in emergency ophthalmology situations. It is aimed at trainees, general ophthalmologists and those with an interest from allied specialties (including specialist nurses) and professions such as optometrists and emergency medicine doctors"-- Provided by publisher.
Identifiers: LCCN 2019034435 (print) | LCCN 2019034436 (ebook) | ISBN 9780367110277 (paperback ; alk. paper) | ISBN 9780367135034 (hardback ; alk. paper) | ISBN 9780429024405 (ebook)
Subjects: MESH: Eye Diseases--therapy | Eye Injuries--therapy | Emergency Treatment | Handbook
Classification: LCC RE48 (print) | LCC RE48 (ebook) | NLM WW 39 | DDC 617.7/025--dc23
LC record available at https://lccn.loc.gov/2019034435
LC ebook record available at https://lccn.loc.gov/2019034436

Visit the Taylor & Francis Web site at
http://www.taylorandfrancis.com

and the CRC Press Web site at
http://www.crcpress.com

The book is dedicated to 'the eye patients of Wales, without whom this book would not be possible.'

Contents

Foreword ix

Introduction xi

Editors xiii

Contributors xv

1. The Red Eye: Basic Algorithm on How to Differentiate Main
   Conditions from Each Other. 1
   Amy-lee Shirodkar

2. Cellulitis and Swelling around One or Both Eyelids 7
   Tina Parmar

3. Watery Eyes 15
   Dana Ahnood

4. Trauma to the Eyelids and Periorbital Region 21
   Abdus Samad Ansari

5. Corneal Ulcers and Contact Lens Keratitis. 29
   Bushra Thajudeen

6. Corneal Defects, Abrasions and Foreign Bodies 37
   Magdalena Popiela

7. Photophobia and Anterior Uveitis 45
   Gwyn Samuel Williams

8. Red Eyes after Cataract Surgery and Other Operations. 53
   Annie See Wah Tung

9. Apparent Sudden Visual Loss: An Essential Approach 59
   Colm McAlinden

10. Flashing Lights and Floaters. 67
    Bhavana Sharma

11. New Haemorrhages in the Vitreous and/or Retina 73
    Tafadzwa Young-Zvandasara

12. There is Something Strange and Unusual at the Back of the Eye 79
    Rhianon Perrott-Reynolds

13. Wavy Lines, Distorted Vision and Blur. 87
    Annie See Wah Tung

14. Vitritis and Posterior Uveitis...95
   Safa Ahmed Elhassan

15. The Painful Eyeball...101
   Alexander Kin Chiang Chiu

16. Retinal Tears and Detachments 107
   Sidath Wijetilleka

17. One or More Bulging Eyes...115
   Derek Kwun-hong Ho

18. Double Vision and New Onset Strabismus in an Adult................123
   Eulee Seow

19. My Baby Has a White Pupil in This Photograph and/or Has a Squint ... 129
   Ryan Davies

20. Non-Accidental Injury 135
   Damien Yeo

21. One or Both Optic Discs are Swollen..............................145
   Tariq Mohammad

22. Headaches and Pain in the Temple 153
   Bhavna Kumari Sharma

23. Managing Ocular Trauma...161
   Bhavin Patel

24. Called to ITU to Examine a Fundus...............................167
   James Potts

25. When There Are Symptoms But it All Looks Totally Normal..........175
   Andrew Want

26. Triage 183
   Amy-lee Shirodkar

27. Summary of Approach...189
   Gwyn Samuel Williams

28. The Moral Ophthalmologist 191
   Gwyn Samuel Williams

Index 195

Foreword

Emergency ophthalmology was, for a long time, considered a 'Cinderella' service. Acute care was historically provided by the most junior members of the eye department, often working with a lack of a consultant support. In response to increasing patient dissatisfaction, the NHS Plan set objectives for all Accident and Emergency services, including those for ophthalmology. The introduction of targets ironically provided the incentive for change and the transformation of acute eye services had begun. Slowly but surely, consultant appointments with sessional commitments to not only deliver but also develop emergency ophthalmic services began to appear across the UK. Their numbers are now such that they have even formed their own society (the British Emergency Eye Care Society [BEECS]) to facilitate best practice and formalise training. The zeitgeist that acute services are as important as any other branch of ophthalmology, and moreover one that demands its own unique skill set, is no better exemplified than the Royal College of Ophthalmologists now recognising emergency ophthalmology as a sub-speciality in its own right. Who would have thought?

Surveys tell us that blindness is feared second only to cancer. It is this fear, real or perceived, that drives patients with ophthalmic symptoms to the emergency department. Disregard whatever preconceptions you may have, the reality is that absolutely anything and everything may be out there lurking in the waiting room. To reliably distinguish the benign and ridiculous from the vision and life threatening, and then instigate appropriate treatment and follow-up, is what makes working in the emergency department as rewarding as it is challenging.

From the very onset of our careers, we are expected to consult and manage patients in the emergency department. The limited ophthalmic knowledge and clinical skills we may have gleaned from medical school hardly prepare us for the task ahead. *The Practical Emergency Ophthalmology Handbook* provides a pragmatic framework of how to assess and manage patients as they present to us in real life. Left to our own devices, breaking down the common presentations into logical algorithms is something we typically only achieve with considerable experience. This publication is, therefore, a timely and useful addition to any trainee' reading list and one which will serve as a useful reference guide as they navigate their way through the emergency department. It is a shame nothing comparable was around when I first set foot in an eye department.

Richard Andrews
Moorfields Eye Hospital

Introduction

Gwyn Samuel Williams and Amy-lee Shirodkar

Every ophthalmologist the world over needs to know how to manage sight-threatening emergencies and may easily be overwhelmed when first confronting the terrifying and dizzying array of horrifying conditions that may be affecting the patient sitting in front of them. But as you begrudgingly approach the seemingly packed out waiting room, the pile of already waiting patients and nurses with queries staring at you wondering what took you so long, you wonder where to start and your anxiety builds. Although we cannot help improve your patient load or hours in a day, we, together with almost every ophthalmology registrar in Wales, have written this book to help arm you with an approach you can implement with each patient you see.

It is a common thing to fear eye casualty sessions and to avoid them as much as possible, with some even contemplating sickness. However, the first step to conquering any problem is to understand it and to break it down into its constituent parts. We have therefore divided the chapters in this book into common presentations that almost every patient attending eye casualty will fall into. While the vast majority of other books out there require the reader to know the diagnosis before being able to look up examination and treatment options, this is a presentation-based book, divided into chapters starting with a logical algorithm that helps guide the inexperienced registrar towards specific diagnoses and therefore plans of action. We hope that by half-knowing a potential plan of action before actually setting eyes on a patient the casualty officer's stress levels will already be reduced and the consultation will therefore be a happier time for both patient and doctor.

There is much to learn when dealing with eye emergencies. Whereas regular clinic patients are easier to deal with as the diagnosis has already been made by others and your decision will be dependent on a much smaller amount of information, for example intraocular pressure in a glaucoma clinic, eye casualty requires a much broader range of possibilities to be simultaneously considered and worked through systematically. It stretches the mind and keeps it fresh. It is the equivalent of Sudoku mind exercises for the ophthalmologist. An ophthalmologist who does regular eye casualty sessions is a better ophthalmologist than one who does not because they know more clinical information, are good communicators and are better at coping with uncertainty. Why is this? Because they have to be. A good eye casualty officer is respected by patients, nurses and colleagues alike. Patients tend more to remember who initially saw them than those who attend to them in follow-up clinics, for good or bad reasons. Nurses know a good eye casualty doctor from a bad one and will seldom withhold their opinion of whom they would rather have working in their clinic, and whom they would not. Some patients will need onward referral to other ophthalmology teams as well, and seniors will quickly develop a sense of which registrars are more or less likely to refer on accurate diagnoses and well managed patients. Your fellow registrars will also learn whom to rely on and who will just dump all their uncertainty and indecision on others. Eye casualty makes an ophthalmologist who they are. It adds drama and excitement to the working week and makes us better, well-rounded clinicians.

There have been a lot of developments in emergency ophthalmology. Various units still refer to eye casualty, as do I, despite it being a dated term. These are usually the same people to refuse to call Accident and Emergency the new-fangled

'Emergency Department', or the even worse 'ED'. Some units have an 'urgent care' or 'Rapid Access Clinic for Eyes', shortened to 'RACE', which is a misnomer when the heaving waiting room and waiting time is taken into account. Others have an Emergency Ophthalmology Suite, and some take the local place name into account for a catchy, or all too often completely unwieldy, acronym. But emergency ophthalmology is changing and is now the newest recognised and fastest growing sub-specialty. There are more consultants being appointed to this sub-specialty than at any other time in history and they even have their own society. There is a scientific rigour and logic being infused like never before to what can easily be described as the most diverse, challenging and rewarding corner of ophthalmology, and this can only be for the benefit of the patients and the profession, as the future-proof pot of generalists begins to re-fill.

So when you are next due in your eye casualty please don't be afraid of the packed out waiting room with patients sitting on coffee tables and standing up, leaning against the rack of patient information leaflets. Don't be stressed when the nurse on spotting you comes running up to tell you about the query retinal detachment that she's just dilated for you and the possible GCA coming in later on. With the knowledge that you are saving sight and changing lives with every consultation, and that each encounter broadens your experience and makes you a better ophthalmologist, and with this book under your arm, take your place in the consulting room with confidence and happiness and make the patients' wait worthwhile. There is no session more rewarding and no session as satisfying. To paraphrase President Kennedy's speech about the Moon – we should choose to do eye casualty not because it is easy but because it is hard; because eye casualty will serve to organise and measure the best of our energies and skills.

This book was written by registrars currently training and undertaking eye casualty sessions. It speaks from experience. We all hope you find it useful and wish you the best of luck in your eye casualty experiences and in your careers as a whole.

Editors

Amy-lee Shirodkar has a special interest in emergency and general ophthalmology. She has completed ophthalmology training in Wales, a TSC in emergency ophthalmology and a Moorfield's fellowship in urgent eye care and general ophthalmology. She is currently the secretary of the British Emergency Eye Care Society (BEECS), a society aimed at improving provision, care and recognition of the sub-speciality. She has a keen interest in ophthalmic training, representing training issues as a trainee representative at college level, undertakes supervision of junior trainees and has developed e-learning material covering aspects of career development as well as surgical and clinical skills. She lives and works in London, enjoying what the city has to bring.

Gwyn Samuel Williams is a consultant ophthalmologist at Singleton Hospital in Swansea with an interest in medical retina and uveitis. He trained in Ophthalmology on the Wales Rotation and completed a Medical Retina fellowship at Moorfields Eye Hospital in London. He is honorary senior lecturer at Swansea University and has a keen interest in writing, reading, and hiking through the beautiful Welsh countryside.

Contributors

Dana Ahnood
Ophthalmic registrar
Wales Rotation

Abdus Samad Ansari
Ophthalmic registrar
Wales Rotation

Alexander Kin Chiang Chiu
Ophthalmic registrar
Wales Rotation

Ryan Davies
Ophthalmic registrar
Wales Rotation

Safa Ahmed Elhassan
Ophthalmic registrar
Wales Rotation

Derek Kwun-hong Ho
Ophthalmic registrar
Wales Rotation

Colm McAlinden
Ophthalmic registrar
Wales Rotation

Tariq Mohammad
Ophthalmic registrar
Wales Rotation

Tina Parmar
Ophthalmic registrar
Wales Rotation

Bhavin Patel
Ophthalmic registrar
Wales Rotation

Rhianon Perrott-Reynolds
Ophthalmic registrar
Wales Rotation

Magdalena Popiela
Ophthalmic registrar
Wales Rotation

James Potts
Ophthalmic registrar
Wales Rotation

Eulee Seow
Ophthalmic registrar
Wales Rotation

Bhavana Sharma
Ophthalmic registrar
Wales Rotation

Bhavna Kumari Sharma
Ophthalmic registrar
Wales Rotation

Amy-lee Shirodkar
Emergency Medicine Fellow at
    Moorfields Eye Hospital
London, England

Bushra Thajudeen
Cornea fellow
Queens Medical Centre
Nottingham, England

Annie See Wah Tung
Ophthalmic registrar
Wales Rotation

Andrew Want
Ophthalmic registrar
Wales Rotation

Sidath Wijetilleka
Ophthalmic registrar
Wales Rotation

Gwyn Samuel Williams
Consultant Ophthalmologist
Singleton Hospital
Sketty, Wales

and

Honorary Senior Lecturer
Swansea University
Swansea, Wales

Damien Yeo
Ophthalmic registrar
Wales Rotation

Tafadzwa Young-Zvandasara
Ophthalmic registrar
Wales Rotation

1   The Red Eye: Basic Algorithm on How to Differentiate Main Conditions from Each Other

Amy-lee Shirodkar

KEY POINTS

1. Appreciate the difference between causes of a red eye that are urgent vs non-urgent
2. Causes of a red eye tend to involve the anterior segment
3. Associated symptoms and history will help localise the problem
4. Lid eversion and checking for corneal sensation are often missed

DIAGRAM OF ALGORITHM

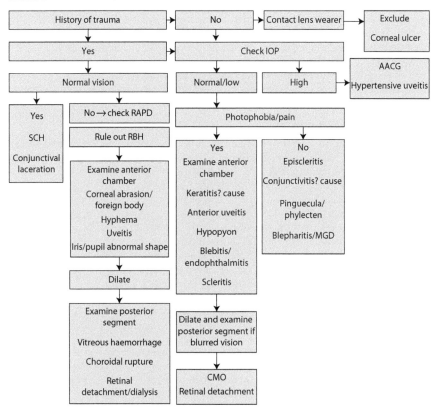

REFERRAL AND PRESENTATION

This is the commonest and least useful presentation of any ophthalmic condition. It can range from the trivial to the potentially blinding and even life-threatening. As such patients may present with a red eye for different reasons and at different time periods depending on a thousand factors ranging from a worry at how they look to a deep seated fear of going blind, with factors such as work, booked holidays or childcare arrangements resulting in great variations as to when a patient with the same condition may present to your department. There may be associated pain, tenderness, photophobia or foreign body sensation – depending on the cause. A red eye might be associated with blurred vision or indeed there may be no visual disability whatsoever. There may be no true emergency, but the eye may just look alarming to friends and family, such as classically with a subconjunctival haemorrhage. Either way, a patient has presented to you with a red eye but you should, through triage, see the true emergencies first: penetrating trauma, acute angle closure glaucoma (AACG) or endophthalmitis for example. Triage is fundamental here more than anywhere.

Knowing the patient's medical history may immediately guide you toward the likely diagnosis, especially if they suffer ocular conditions that have a high risk of recurring such as uveitis, marginal keratitis and herpetic disease for example, or have recently had eye surgery. Systemic conditions with known ocular associations should guide thought processes such that patients with rheumatoid arthritis for example may be more likely to present with corneal melting and scleritis than a patient who has osteoarthritis. Taking a drug history may shine the light on a reason for extensive subconjunctival haemorrhage such as an anticoagulant or use of a topical medication causing allergy. Other important questions to ask in the history include: contact lens wear, potential causes of trauma, recent surgery, previous ocular conditions and past medical history including atopy.

DIFFERENTIAL DIAGNOSIS

The eye may appear red for two reasons: haemorrhage or inflammation. Haemorrhage can appear spontaneously such as with subconjunctival haemorrhage after trauma (blunt, penetrating or iatrogenic) or secondary to infections such as viral conjunctivitis. A red, injected eye with varying pain may be due to inflammation or infection of one or more components of the eye. There are two main ways to sort out the causes of a red eye in your mind. One method is to classify causes by anatomy (see Table 1.1) the second by severity and likelihood of permanent visual injury (see Table 1.2). Ultimately there are only a handful of true ophthalmic emergencies that will cause permanent sight loss if not treated urgently: orbital cellulitis, retrobulbar haemorrhage, AACG, globe disruption (through trauma or corneoscleral melting) and endophthalmitis. The other eye conditions can be classified as urgent or non-urgent depending on the probability of causing permanent irreversible blindness.

CLINICAL EXAMINATION

Begin by measuring the visual acuity for both eyes. If the patient is in too much pain to continue, consider dimming the lights or using topical anaesthetic. Bear in mind that if it is a nurse and not yourself measuring the acuity that Snellen charts in particular, and all acuity tests to a lesser degree, are inherently poor testing modalities and a whole host of different results may be obtained depending on the level of patience present, cooperativeness of the patient or even something as simple as possession of the correct pair of distance glasses. If a visual acuity does not make sense in light of your own examination have a low threshold to retest the acuity yourself. This sort of error is not uncommon.

Table 1.1: **Causes of Red Eye Diagnoses Depending on Affected Area**

Affected Area	Causes of Red Eye
Eyelids	Cellulitis – orbital, preseptal Blepharitis Molluscum Herpes zoster ophthalmicus Entropion, ectropion, trichiasis
Conjunctiva	SCH Conjunctivitis – infective, allergic, autoimmune
Sclera/episclera	Scleritis, episcleritis
Cornea	Keratitis Infective – viral, bacterial, acanthamoeba Inflammatory – marginal keratitis, peripheral ulcerative keratitis, superior limbic keratitis Corneal abrasion, erosion, exposure Neuropathic causes of abrasion or ulceration
Anterior chamber	Uveitis, hyphema
Raised IOP	Glaucoma – AACG, secondary causes
Lens	Phacolytic, phacomorphic, phacoanaphylactic glaucoma
Others	Carotid cavernous fistula, malignant lesions, retrobulbar haemorrhage
Trauma	Laceration – eyelids, cornea, sclera, IOFB

Table 1.2: **Triage of Red Eye Depending on Cause**

Emergency	Urgent	Non-Urgent
Acute angle closure glaucoma	Uveitis	Conjunctivitis
Endophthalmitis	Keratitis	Chalazion
Orbital cellulitis	Scleritis	Dry eyes/Blepharitis
Disrupted globe integrity – Corneal perforation (ulcer, melt, trauma) Necrotising scleritis Trauma		SCH
Retrobulbar haemorrhage		Episcleritis
		Conjunctivitis

General observation will highlight signs of trauma or facial pathology. The stoop of a person as they enter the room may indicate ankylosing spondylitis and thus a higher probability of uveitis. Make a note of anything unusual or out of the ordinary.

Perform slit lamp examination beginning with examining the eyelids, including position, function and never forget lid eversion to look for follicles, papillae or foreign body. A cotton bud can help you here (see Figure 1.1). Identify whether the eyeball is tender to palpation and the location, distribution and layer of involved blood vessels that are inflamed. Differentiate a red eye due to bleeding, inflammation or both.

Look at the cornea for foreign objects, opacities, infections or haze. Check for corneal sensation, then stain using fluorescein. Remember to examine the superior cornea covered by the upper lid. Measure any defects – epithelial or deeper and any infiltrates using the graticule on the slit lamp and document this clearly (see Figure 1.2).

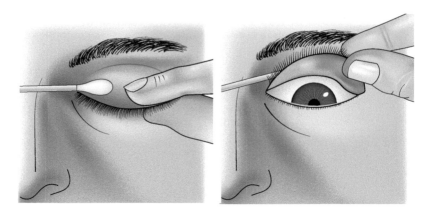

Figure 1.1 How to evert the upper eyelid using a cotton bud.

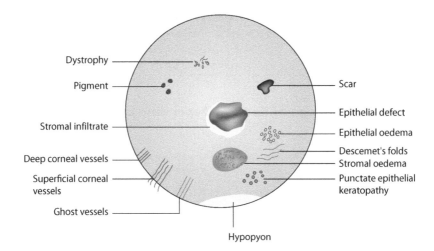

Figure 1.2 How to document surface pathology of the eye.

View the anterior chamber for white cells, hyphema or hypopyon and note the depth. Measure the intraocular pressure (IOP). If the IOP is raised perform gonioscopy in both eyes. In some cases an I-CARE tonometer may be suitable, especially in children.

Note any iris changes – colour, shape, position, symmetry and size. It is vital to assess pupillary reactions before dilating drops are used. Make a note of lens status, position and presence or absence of cataract.

After ruling out angle closure and examining the pupil appropriately, dilate the pupil to examine the posterior segment for involvement of inflammatory diseases, causes of neovascular glaucoma and additional sites of potential trauma. Perform a dilated examination to identify causes of reduced vision when the anterior segment media are clear. Consider performing a B-scan if you cannot view the fundus – be gentle if suspecting a penetrating injury. Dilate all cases of anterior uveitis. In fact have a very low threshold for dilating all patients; if in doubt, dilate.

Examine surgical sites for loose sutures, infection, inflammation or dehiscence.

INVESTIGATIONS

Follow local protocols where they exist.

Investigations are useful for diagnosing and differentiating causes of infections:

- Swabs – Viral, bacterial and Chlamydial can all be taken for signs of conjunctivitis or cellulitis when the cause is not evident from the history or the clinical findings.
- Corneal scrape of a corneal ulcer helps to identify organisms and direct treatment for speedy resolution. Do not commence topical antibiotic treatment until a scrape has been undertaken!
- Where available, arrange confocal microscopy to identify acanthamoeba cysts
- Anterior chamber and vitreous tap/biopsy would be analysed to identify organisms causing infectious uveitis or endophthalmitis.

Imaging is important to view the integrity of the globe, orbit and facial bones in cases of severe cellulitis, trauma or retained intraocular foreign body. CT is best at looking at bony structures and MRI is best for looking at the soft tissues of the orbit or brain, though obviously this is contraindicated in cases of suspected metallic intraocular foreign body.

Systemic blood tests may be required to identify associations and monitor progression for infectious, autoimmune and inflammatory conditions when scleritis, uveitis or cellulitis is diagnosed.

Intraocular samples are required when endophthalmitis is suspected and systemic work up for endogenous cases. Blood culture is also indicated if a patient presents with suspected endogenous endophthalmitis.

DIAGNOSIS

Diagnosis will come from a combination of history taking and examination and occasionally be apparent only after undertaking investigations. A list of causes of a red eye are shown in Table 1.1 and in the algorithm above. The most important aspect is to separate potential sight and life threatening diagnoses from those that are more mundane.

MANAGEMENT

Some causes of a red eye need no treatment including subconjunctival haemorrhage, bacterial and viral conjunctivitis (without corneal involvement). Others require specific regimes according to local guidelines. See individual chapters for further information. Essentially antibiotics and/or antivirals are given for infections and steroids for non-infectious causes of inflammation. Mistreatment or undertreatment of either is a major pitfall. Follow local protocols where they exist.

Documentation is key for medico legal issues and to better inform the next person of the patient's story. Note the time and date of your examination, and clearly document your name. Consider taking photographs to document trauma and the extent of corneal or eyelid pathology.

If you find yourself in doubt about a diagnosis or how to perform an investigation or treatment, always ask for senior support. This will ensure timely management and treatment for potentially sight-threatening conditions. This principle is the same regardless of how busy the clinic is, or how close you are to the end of your shift.

Remember to manage the patient holistically, identifying safeguarding issues and addressing patient concerns where appropriate. This is also true of explaining the nature of the treatment and the importance of compliance. Leaflets can be useful but are no substitute for a proper explanation.

FOLLOW UP

Not all causes of a red eye will need to be reviewed again and those that do may vary from requiring next day review, one week review or two weekly review or even longer. As the evidence base for emergency ophthalmology is sparse, you will learn through teaching and experience the duration of follow up for each case and which conditions you can safely discharge. Be tactful and bring back cases when specialty consultants are around for sub-specialist input.

Life threatening associations with a red eye are rare however be mindful to check or refer the patient urgently to their GP for: blood pressure and INR in subconjunctival haemorrhage, systemic inflammation in corneal melts, infections in endogenous endophthalmitis and other bodily injuries with trauma.

If discharging patients, educate those with recurrent or preventable diagnoses to stop them coming back or presenting late! And always play safe and remind your patients to come back if their symptoms get worse. Use informative patient leaflets where available.

To gain experience always read up around your cases and follow up your own patients and review their progress and again; if in doubt always ask for senior help if unsure. It is sadly not uncommon for eye casualty officers to bring difficult patients back to see a colleague during another session so that they need not face the uncertainty of not knowing what is going on. This causes confusion and delay.

PITFALLS

1. Poor history taking fails to identify associated activities or medial history. Always think contact lens.
2. Forgetting to check corneal sensation.
3. Failure to evert the eyelids. Occasionally you will be surprised at what you might find.
4. Failure to identify and treat the real emergencies in a timely manner – AACG, endophthalmitis, and penetrating injuries.
5. Poor documentation.
6. Failure to involve senior colleagues early and not asking for help.

FURTHER READING

Denniston A., P. Murray *Oxford Handbook of Ophthalmology*. Oxford University Press, 2018.

2   Cellulitis and Swelling around One or Both Eyelids

Tina Parmar

KEY POINTS
1. Sight and life threatening causes must be recognised as soon as possible
2. Have a low threshold for initiating aggressive treatment in young, elderly, immunocompromised or uncontrolled diabetic patients
3. Have a multidisciplinary approach to the management of eyelid swelling
4. Bilateral cases of pre-septal or orbital cellulitis in a healthy person warrant further investigation

DIAGRAM OF ALGORITHM

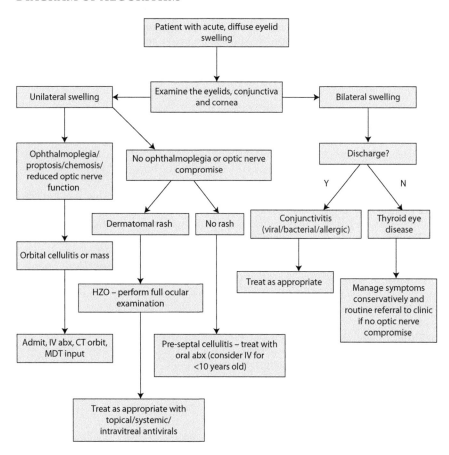

N.B. This is clearly not an exhaustive list for the causes of an acute presentation of diffuse eyelid swelling. Be aware that unilateral conditions may rarely become bilateral and that typical bilateral conditions may be asymmetric.

REFERRAL AND PRESENTATION

There are many causes of eyelid swelling and your most important task is to determine whether it is a sight, or worse still, a life-threatening condition.

Eyelid swelling can present in patients of any age, be acute or chronic, unilateral or bilateral, affect the upper or lower lid (or both), be diffuse or well defined, painful or non-painful, tense or boggy. Patients may complain of reduced vision due to mechanical compression, ptosis, or optic nerve compromise or diplopia when associated with muscular or orbital involvement.

Always remember to have a low threshold for serious pathology in the very young, elderly, diabetic or immunocompromised patient. Check for systemic features including vital signs: temperature, blood pressure, heart rate and blood sugar levels as well as other ocular associations including discharge, ophthalmoplegia or surrounding skin features.

DIFFERENTIAL DIAGNOSIS

It is important to differentiate between the aetiology of lid swelling as treatment differs. Antibiotics would be required for an infective cellulitis, but steroids would be used to treat idiopathic orbital inflammation for example. A list of differentials for eyelid swelling can be categorised as unilateral or bilateral to aid logical thinking.

Unilateral eyelid swelling: Unilateral eyelid swelling may be diffuse or discrete.

A diffuse, tense lid swelling is likely to be of an infectious aetiology. The most important thing to do in these cases is to determine whether this is a case of pre-septal or orbital cellulitis. Have a low index of suspicion of orbital involvement in children as the source is often the paranasal air sinuses, which can lead to abscess formation within the orbit or worse still, spread to the brain and meninges causing risk to life and thus should not be missed or under-treated.

Other important infections include necrotising fasciitis and mucormycosis, both rare, but progress rapidly with devastating consequences. Orbital inflammatory diseases mimic orbital cellulitis, can be recurrent and associated with systemic conditions.

Trauma is another cause of eyelid swelling, retrobulbar haemorrhage the most emergent, but it is usually quite apparent from the history and other features such as cuts, bruises or fractures. It is important to remember that base of skull fractures may present with 'racoon eyes' (see Figure 2.1) so ensure you check for other signs such as Battle's sign, CSF rhinorrhoea and cranial nerve palsies. Trauma is covered in further detail in a later chapter.

Discrete lesions may be due to chalazia, hordeolum, pyogenic granuloma, neurofibromas, skin cancers and so forth. Inflamed or infected lesions may cause superimposed diffuse eyelid swelling, with tenderness over the responsible lesion, including Dacryocyctitis causing cellulitis and pain over nasolacrimal duct.

Swelling emerging from the superotemporal aspect of the orbit (producing the classic S-shaped ptosis) should raise suspicion of a lacrimal gland swelling, the causes of which may be either infectious such as dacryoadenitis, inflammatory or neoplastic (see Figure 2.2).

Bilateral eyelid swelling: Commonly, bilateral eyelid swelling is usually due to a more benign cause and often associated with an allergen or an infective conjunctivitis.

A history of exposure to a new pet, a bee sting, new medication or experimenting with different cuisines or cosmetics may point towards an allergic cause, in which

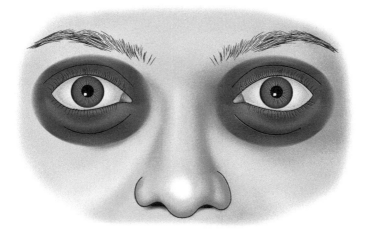

Figure 2.1 'Racoon eyes' typically seen in skull base fracture.

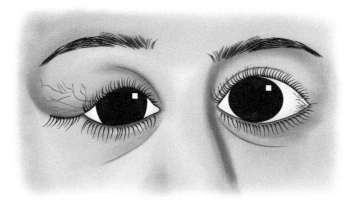

Figure 2.2 Typical S-shaped upper eyelid swelling seen in lacrimal gland swelling.

case do not forget to ask about swelling of the lips or throat when triaging. Sticky or watery discharge suggests conjunctivitis, which can produce quite an impressive swollen eyelid in viral conjunctivitis.

Check the thyroid status of the patient as unilateral or bilateral eyelid swelling and erythema is often a subtle feature of thyroid eye disease. A flare up of blepharitis may also be responsible for an acute unilateral or bilateral swelling of the eyelids, but is often accompanied with soreness, itchy eyes, photophobia and possibly discharge.

CLINICAL EXAMINATION

It is always important to take a thorough clinical history and perform a brief general inspection of the patient before looking at the eyes, as helpful signs may be overlooked. Mobility problems may indicate an inflammatory pathology, if the patient appears systemically unwell then an infectious cause is likely, and systemic features of thyroid dysfunction may point towards thyroid eye disease.

Face and skin:

- Inspect for swelling, for example the lips (allergy) or the glands (such as mumps or sarcoid in parotid gland swelling).

- Check for pre-auricular lymph nodes, which are often inflamed in viral conditions.

- The skin should be closely examined. Eczema is often associated with atopic keratoconjunctivitis and in rosacea, with blepharitis being closely linked; a dermatomal skin rash is likely to be Herpes Zoster but this may be subtle in early stages.

- Check for wounds on the skin, as they may be the source of an infection. Skin around the eyelids have few adhesions to underlying tissues making them more prone to oedematous swelling than other areas of the face. The offending lesion therefore may be some distance from the eyes so thoroughly check the scalp and face.

Pay particular attention to patients that are immunocompromised, uncontrolled diabetics, cancer sufferers, obese, alcoholic or intravenous drug users, as they all carry a greater risk of necrotising fasciitis and Mucormycosis – two rapidly progressive, flesh-destroying conditions, as well as erysipelas; a superficial dermal and lymphatic infection caused by *Streptococcus pyogenes*. Greyish-blue or black necrotic lesions around the skin or nose are signs to look out for in these conditions. The tell-tale signs of herpes simplex must also be looked for.

Optic nerve function: Assess visual acuity with and without pinhole. Lid swelling may cause warping of the cornea resulting in reduced vision due to refractive errors. Colour vision is also essential to check the optic nerve function as the optic nerve may be compromised by post-septal conditions. Consider performing visual fields to confrontation or formal perimetry if suspicious of orbital involvement.

Extraocular movements: Assess and document restriction and diplopia. Many patients who are merely in discomfort, however, will complain that they are unable to look at extreme gazes often a limitation due to pain rather than true mechanical restriction that occurs in the presence of an abscess.

Proptosis: Should be measured by exophthalmometry, and retropulsion for signs of a tense orbit. If one eye can be pushed back into the orbit more easily than the other this is valuable information that may indicate trouble within the orbit.

Eyelids: Take a closer look at the eyelids with a magnified view, paying particular attention to the eyelid margins. Check for any discrete lumps, bumps or skin changes and always evert the eyelids to check for papillae, follicles or foreign bodies. Look at the bulbar conjunctiva, areas hidden underneath the eyelids and over muscle insertion points for injection, chemosis or other lesions.

The rest of the eye: After this move on to examining the eye itself. Assess corneal exposure, sensation and integrity; look for any ulcers or infiltrates, such as subepithelial infiltrates seen in adenoviral conjunctivitis. Examine the anterior chamber for inflammation, then the intraocular pressure, which may be asymmetrical with a collection or inflammation within the orbit or muscles. Then check the pupils for a relative afferent pupillary defect (RAPD) before dilating to examine the fundus, paying particular attention to the appearance of the optic nerve and the presence or absence of choroidal folds.

INVESTIGATIONS

The extent to which you investigate depends on the findings of your history and examination.

Swabs: Take bacterial and/or viral swabs for conjunctival discharge, secretions or weeping skin lesions.

Blood tests: Consider infectious and inflammatory markers (see uveitis section), thyroid function tests (TFTs) and thyroid autoantibodies (anti-thyroid peroxidase antibodies (anti-TPO antibodies), thyrotropin receptor antibodies (TRAbs) and thyroglobulin antibodies), and blood cultures if there is systemic upset. Hereditary angioedema is a rare cause for eyelid, lip and tongue swelling which is associated with a low level of C1-esterase inhibitor. Angioedema may also be the result of taking ACE inhibitors.

Ocular investigations: Perform formal perimetry if there is suspicion of optic nerve dysfunction. Ocular ultrasound by a can be helpful to identify abnormal extraocular muscles or retrobulbar pathology, if performed by a competent ultrasonographer, otherwise stick to CT or MRI.

Imaging: If there are any signs or proptosis, diminished ocular motility or optic nerve dysfunction, an urgent high-resolution CT scan of the brain, orbit and sinuses with/without contrast must be organised. CT scans of children should be discussed ideally with a senior colleague as the child may need sedation. Be specific about what it is you are concerned about on the request form; the more information that you provide to your neuroradiologist, the more you will get back from them. If the CT is not fruitful but you still suspect intraorbital involvement, consider an MRI scan (with STIR sequencing for thyroid eye disease).

DIAGNOSIS

Now you must piece together the findings from your history, examination and investigations to complete the puzzle, though do not waste time and delay treatment by waiting for the results of your investigation, especially in critical situations. This is where your clinical acumen comes into its own, though always follow local protocols where available.

Cellulitis: In a bacterial cellulitis, there will be a tense, warm, erythematous swelling of either the upper, lower or both eyelids. It is uncommon to have a bilateral pre-septal or orbital cellulitis, and if this is the case, the patient should be investigated further for causes of immunosuppression. Features that distinguish a pre-septal from an orbital cellulitis include grossly reduced visual acuity, proptosis, chemosis, ophthalmoplegia and optic nerve dysfunction, expressed via reduced fields, colour vision and the presence of an RAPD. There is a myth that the presence of a demarcation line at the border of the orbit is useful in differentiating pre-septal from orbital cellulitis, but this is unreliable at best and misleading at worst.

MANAGEMENT

The management of eyelid swelling is obviously dependant on the cause. Rule out TED complications and refer potentially malignant lesions urgently. Other benign causes of lid swelling can be reviewed in a subspecialty or general outpatient clinic.

Pre-septal cellulitis: If a patient is referred with a confident diagnosis of a pre-septal cellulitis, they rarely need to be seen by an ophthalmologist and can be treated with a course of oral co-amoxiclav or flucloxacillin (or erythromycin if penicillin allergic) and advise warm compress for cases secondary to chalazia/stye. *Staphylococcus aureus* and *Streptococcus pyogenes* are typical microbes responsible for causing pre-septal cellulitis. As mentioned earlier, have a low threshold for seeing and admitting children for intravenous (IV) therapy, especially for children under 9, who are more at risk of developing orbital cellulitis, with whom the child should be under joint care with the paediatric team for close monitoring. You may also consider admitting vulnerable patients such as diabetics, immunocompromised patients, alcoholics, those not responding to oral antibiotics or those who are systemically very unwell. Use your clinical acumen and follow local protocols and discuss with your senior.

Orbital cellulitis: Patients diagnosed with orbital cellulitis need to be admitted and IV antibiotics commenced straight away. Infectious organisms commonly include *Staphylococcus aureus, Streptococcus pneumoniae, Streptococcus pyogenes* and *Haemophilus influenzae,* which can spread into the orbit from skin infections, paranasal sinuses or haematologically.

You should follow local guidelines for the treatment of orbital cellulitis or get microbiology advice.

- Common treatment for children is IV flucloxacillin, ceftazidime and metronidazole. The patient should be apyrexial for 4 days and then they can be switched to oral therapy for 1–3 weeks.

- Draw around the affected area with a skin marker on admission or better still, ask a family member to take daily photographs on their smartphone so progression can be easily monitored.

- Take swabs and blood cultures where indicated.

- Don't forget to inform the on call consultant (or oculoplastic/paediatric-ophthalmologist) if you admit a patient under their care.

- Severe cases may need review more than once in 24 hours, senior review should occur within 12–14 hours of admission and involve ENT if the sinuses are involved.

- If abscess formation is evident on CT imaging, it is essential to get your ENT colleagues involved, as they will be very helpful with draining the abscess and exploring the paranasal sinuses.

- Remember to prescribe regular lubricants for those at risk of exposure keratopathy secondary to proptosis and IOP lowering medication for raised intraocular pressure.

Rapid progression of cellulitis, not responding to IV therapy should prompt you to explore further. The presence of bullae, ecchymosis or necrosis should start ringing alarm bells (necrotising fasciitis or mucormycosis) and will need urgent imaging (CT or ocular ultrasound) for locules of gas and urgent surgical debridement with the help of the orbital and/or maxilla-facial teams as deemed appropriate.

Complications of orbital cellulitis, although rare, include subperiosteal abscess formation (often involving the medial wall of the orbit), brain abscess, meningitis, endophthalmitis, central retinal vein occlusions and cavernous sinus thrombosis.

FOLLOW UP

Pre-septal cellulitis: If the diagnosis is simply a pre-septal cellulitis in a young, healthy adult, then it is reasonable to discharge the patient with treatment and SOS advice. Alternatively you can call them back in 5–7 days to check their response. I will usually always call back children unless you are certain that you can rely on the parents to bring the child back if the condition is not resolving as expected, and beware of large chalazia obstructing vision in a small child. If you feel that the case is severe but not severe enough to be admitted, recalling the patient for assessment after 48 hours of oral antibiotics is a safe and reasonable option.

Any patient that you admit must have a daily review, even if they are under the care of another team such as paediatrics or ENT; remember they are under joint care and communicate your findings and management plan clearly.

Once discharged, I would see again in 5–7 days by oculoplastic or paediatric-ophthalmology colleagues. You may discharge the patient once the infection is completely resolved; however, if the cellulitis is thought to be due to a blockage in the lacrimal drainage system (i.e. secondary to a dacrocystitis), then the patient needs to be referred to the oculoplastics team for assessment and consideration of surgery such as probing or a dacryorhinocystotomy (DCR).

PITFALLS

1. The biggest pitfall is not recognising the signs of serious conditions and initiating treatment in a timely manner. If the assessment of the eye and orbit is not thorough, then signs can easily be missed.
2. Sometimes it may be difficult to examine non-cooperative patients but this is not an excuse to miss signs. Be patient with your patient. If a child is becoming frustrated, maybe send them away for half an hour and then try to reassess. If it still feels like an impossible task, ask a senior for advice.
3. We've all learnt from our days at medical school the importance of working in a multidisciplinary team. Be sure to involve others and use their skills. This may include the orthoptics, paediatrics, ENT, maxillofacial, microbiology, neuroradiology, endocrine (for thyroid eye disease), general medical or care of the elderly, or even ITU with unstable patients.
4. Have a low threshold for performing CTs in the young.

FURTHER READING

Bowling B. *Kanski's Clinical Ophthalmology: A Clinical Approach*; 8th ed. Elsevier, 2016. Chapters 1,3, pp. 2–62, 78–117.

Witmer M. Unravelling the difficult diagnosis of dacryoadenitis. *Review of Ophthalmology*. 2009; 26(8).

3 Watery Eyes

Dana Ahnood

KEY POINTS

1. Watery eyes can be an emergency in the context of acute dacryocystitis or severe ocular surface disease.
2. If you are worried about a tumour as a cause of nasolacrimal duct obstruction, speak to the oculoplastic team and consider CT imaging.
3. Perform syringing and probing if nasolacrimal duct obstruction is suspected. This requires a good amount of practice under supervision to get really expert at this.

DIAGRAM OF ALGORITHM

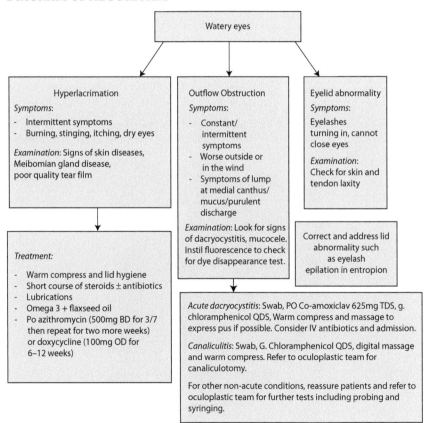

Watery eyes

Hyperlacrimation

Symptoms:

- Intermittent symptoms
- Burning, stinging, itching, dry eyes

Examination: Signs of skin diseases, Meibomian gland disease, poor quality tear film

Treatment:

- Warm compress and lid hygiene
- Short course of steroids ± antibiotics
- Lubrications
- Omega 3 + flaxseed oil
- Po azithromycin (500mg BD for 3/7 then repeat for two more weeks) or doxycycline (100mg OD for 6–12 weeks)

Outflow Obstruction

Symptoms:

- Constant/ intermittent symptoms
- Worse outside or in the wind
- Symptoms of lump at medial canthus/ mucus/purulent discharge

Examination: Look for signs of dacryocystitis, mucocele. Instil fluorescence to check for dye disappearance test.

Acute dacryocystitis: Swab, PO Co-amoxiclav 625mg TDS, g. chloramphenicol QDS, Warm compress and massage to express pus if possible. Consider IV antibiotics and admission.

Canaliculitis: Swab, G. Chloramphenicol QDS, digital massage and warm compress. Refer to oculoplastic team for canaliculotomy.

For other non-acute conditions, reassure patients and refer to oculoplastic team for further tests including probing and syringing.

Eyelid abnormality

Symptoms:

Eyelashes turning in, cannot close eyes

Examination: Check for skin and tendon laxity

Correct and address lid abnormality such as eyelash epilation in entropion

REFERRAL AND PRESENTATION

Watery eyes, termed epiphora, may be the least of your worries on a Friday afternoon, but to the patient, epiphora can be disabling. Epiphora occurs when there is the slightest imbalance of tear production and absorption and can occur due to problems with any part of the lacrimal apparatus causing increased tear production.

Patients may present to the urgent eye care service with or without associated symptoms such as foreign body sensation, pain, photophobia or discharge. The majority of patients suffering from epiphora are cases of innocuous, common causes managed in eye casualty to include foreign body, keratitis, malpositioned eyelashes/lid and conjunctivitis.

Conditions causing acute blockage of the nasolacrimal segment that would need early intervention include tumour or infection. Chronic epiphora should be re-directed to outpatient clinics, and advice on how to manage secondary causes, such as lid disease, should be instigated.

DIFFERENTIAL DIAGNOSIS

Differential diagnoses of a watery eye can be classified into three main categories:

Hyperlacrimation: The overproduction of normal tears may occur secondary to ocular surface disease and conjunctivitis. The overproduction of poor quality tears, sometimes confusingly termed 'dry eyes' can be caused by anything from drugs and radiotherapy to autoimmune diseases such as Sjögren's syndrome or meibomian gland dysfunction. It often confuses patients in this situation that an ocular lubricant can actually help with their watery eyes.

Eyelid malposition: If a regular amount of normal quality tears are produced this can still lead to watering if the eyelid impedes its flow through to the puncta. This can be due to ectropion, entropion, lagophthalmos and any punctual abnormalities.

Nasolacrimal duct obstruction: This may occur at any point from the punctum to the nose (see Figure 3.1) due to infection, inflammation, compression or infiltration.

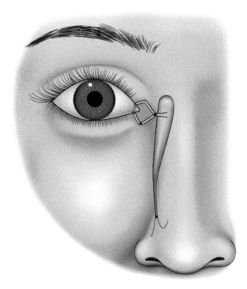

Figure 3.1 A diagram of the nasolacrimal drainage apparatus and the possible sites of blockage.

CLINICAL EXAMINATION

Before getting anywhere near the eye, ask yourself if the patient is systemically unwell. If so, ask the nursing staff to measure the blood pressure, pulse and temperature as a bare minimum. Only then is it safe and appropriate to examine the face. Start from outside and work your way in towards the eye.

Face: First inspect the patient's face for rosacea, acne, eczema or any other skin diseases. Look for facial asymmetry indicative of facial nerve palsy which may be contributing to a paralytic ectropion or lagophthalmos which can cause a watery eye due to corneal exposure.

Eyelids: Then go in further and examine the eyelids themselves. Are the eyelids in a normal position and do they have a normal contour? Are there any lumps, cysts or notches in or around the eyelids? If so these may be irritating the ocular surface with subsequent watery eyes. Ask the patient to close their eyes gently, then forcefully observing for how much of the eye is exposed and documenting the measurement, presence of a Bell's phenomenon (the eye rolling upwards so the cornea is covered by the upper lid) and for signs of an entropion. Check for eyelid laxity by stretching the medial and lateral canthal tendons. Lower eyelid laxity can be demonstrated if the lid can be pulled away from the globe by more than 6 mm.

Eyelashes: Using the slit lamp look for evidence of malpositioned eyelashes abraiding the cornea (trichiasis, dystichiasis) and for signs of blepharitis or meibomian gland dysfunction.

Conjunctiva: Next examine all aspects of the bulbar conjunctiva by asking the patient to look up, down, left and right. Don't forget to lift the upper lid when patient is looking down and to lift the lower lid down when patient is looking up. There might be a foreign body or any other matter that is irritating the eye. Evert the eyelids and look at the subtarsal conjunctiva for evidence of follicles, papillae, foreign body or even concretions which may give a clue as to the cause of the watery eyes.

Nasolacrimal system: Start with the punctum, which should be positioned at the conjunctival tear lake. Look for evidence of stenosis, inflammation, bleeding, pus/ discharge, granules or obstruction. Look and feel for a mass or inflammation arising in the medial canthus, which may be due to acute dacryocystitis, a mucocele, or a tumour; compare both sides for symmetry.

Tear film: Finally examine the tear film and quality. The presence of a foamy tear film near the lid margins, mucous and debris indicates tear inadequacy and inflammation. A tear break up time of less than 10 seconds is abnormal. This is measured by instilling fluorescein 2% and observing the tear film through the slit lamp with a cobalt blue filter. Once the patient blinks, measure the time taken for the first dry spot to appear on the cornea. Presence of a dry spot in less than 10 second suggests a tear film abnormality.

INVESTIGATIONS

Most patients don't require radiological investigations in acute settings; removal of the offending stimulant is cure enough. However, the following can be useful:

1. CT imaging is invaluable in assessing the bone and soft tissues around the nasolacrimal system including identifying sinus abnormalities and tumours.

2. Dacryocystography (DCG) assesses the anatomy of nasolacrimal system using CT imaging with the aid of contrast. Obstruction to the flow of contrast injected via the punctum into the NL system can be visualised on sequential images for both eyes.

3. Scintigraphy: This is a radionuclide test that is useful when suspecting functional obstruction.

If an infection is suspected such as canaliculitis or dacryocystitis it is useful to take swabs of any fluid or pus in the conjunctival sac or around the punctum and send them for microbiological analysis.

DIAGNOSIS

You should be able to clinically diagnose most acute causes of epiphora. However, when suspecting nasolacrimal duct obstruction, lacrimal syringing is essential to establish the level of obstruction within the system. This does not need to be routinely done at eye casualty, but you may find it a useful skill in some circumstances.

There are three main tests used to evaluate watery eyes.

1. *Dye disappearance test:* This involves instilling fluorescein 2% in the inferior conjunctiva. After 5 minutes using a cobalt blue light check for stagnation of the fluorescein 2% in the tear lake suggestive of a non-functioning nasolacrimal system.

2. *Primary Jones test:* Immediately after the disappearance dye test (5 minutes post fluorescence instillation), place a cotton bud at the inferior turbinate of the nose. Absence of fluorescein on the cotton bud suggests a poorly functioning nasolacrimal system.

3. *Secondary Jones test:* When no dye is recovered in the primary Jones test this test can be performed next. This test is mainly intended to examine what is recovered from the inferior turbinate following punctual irrigation with normal saline. If fluorescein is recovered from the inferior turbinate, then a partial blockage is likely. If only normal saline is recovered, this suggests a partial or a functional blockage of the canaliculi. Finally, if no fluid is recovered from the nose then a total obstruction is likely.

Syringing is a procedure to show patency of the nasolacrimal system; the steps are as follows:

- Remove residual fluorescein by irrigating the inferior conjunctiva with normal saline.

- Instil topical anaesthesia

- Assemble a lacrimal cannula on to a 2.5 mL syringe filled with normal saline

- Pull the lower lid laterally to tauten the skin and straighten the canaliculus (see Figure 3.2).

- Push some saline into the system and tell the patient to let you know when they can taste the salty solution

- Look for fluid/pus/blood regurgitating back through either punctum.

The lower and upper canaliculi are in turn irrigated. Note what is regurgitated back through the upper and lower puncti. Regurgitation of pus suggests a mucocele, whereas regurgitation of some fluorescein suggests that fluorescein had entered the sac and therefore the obstruction is either partial or distal to the nasoclacrimal sac.

If you find the punctum is too small, use a punctual dilator or the end of the punctual plug to gently enlarge the punctum. Then use a punctal wire and advance it through the canaliculi until a 'stop' is felt.

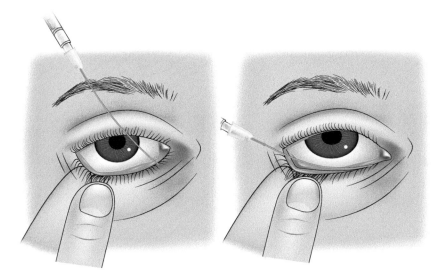

Figure 3.2   Preparing the lower eyelid and punctum for syringing.

- If a hard stop is felt, then it is likely that you are at the level of lacrimal bone (medial aspect of the lacrimal sac) and that the proximal nasolacrimal system until then is patent.
- If the cannula stops at a soft spot, then obstruction at the level of canaliculus or opening of the common canaliculus is common.

The secondary Jones test plus syringing and probing will give you the most information about the nature of the nasolacrimal duct obstruction.

MANAGEMENT

Management of epiphora is targeted at treating the cause.

Dry eyes: Watery eyes worse in windy weather or due to simple dry eyes can be managed with topical lubricants; it is not an ocular emergency and is normal. If you suspect hyperlacrimation then treatment should target the cause. For example, lubricants for dry eyes, warm compress, lid hygiene or a course of oral azithromycin or doxycycline for blepharitis.

Eyelid position: If there is an abnormality of eyelid position, then corrective treatment involves a combination of both medical and surgical treatments. For example, for a patient with a lower lid entropion this may involve epilation of offending eyelashes and taping the lower eyelid down whilst awaiting entropion repair surgery. It is always important to beware of corneal ulcers in these patients. Involve oculoplastics early

Puntum: Treatment of punctual stenosis involves routine referral to your oculoplastic team for consideration of punctoplasty.

Dacryocystitis: If you suspect nasolacrimal obstruction, then an acute infection such as a dacryocystitis needs to be excluded. Treatment of dacryocystitis involves oral co-amoxiclav 625 mg TDS, G. chloramphenicol QDS, warm compress and massage of the lacrimal sac to encourage expression of the pus from the sac. Mark the area of cellulitis (or take photographs) as they need to be reviewed in 24–48 hours to ensure cellulitis is not worsening, but is beginning to improve. Consider admission and IV antibiotics with cases of severe cellulitis. If dacryocystitis is present but the abscess is not 'pointing' it is prudent to leave things be; only incise an abscess if it was going to burst spontaneously.

Canaliculitis: Presents with acute or chronic inflammation around the canaliculi and adjacent lid margin with pus visible on manipulation of the area. Treatment involves warm compresses and topical chloramphenicol in the eye casualty setting, but the patient should be referred to oculoplastics for surgical canaliculotomy to remove concretions, sulphur granules and discharge. The organism responsible for canaliculitis is classically actinomyces iraelii.

Nasolacrimal duct obstruction: With no evidence of acute infection or tumour, this condition will need syringing and irrigation in the outpatient clinic. Trauma to the eyelids and nasolacrimal system causing epiphora is covered elsewhere.

FOLLOW UP

Follow up will depend on the cause of the watery eye. If in doubt, discuss the patient with the oculoplastic team in the presence of a healthy cornea. If you suspect a nasolacrimal duct obstruction, refer to a lacrimal clinic for syringing and probing. Patients with resolving dacryocystitis need to be followed up in outpatient oculoplastic clinics for consideration of dacryocystorhinostomy (DCR). Eyelid malposition, causing corneal exposure or trauma require urgent oculoplastic review for surgical correction.

If you suspect ocular surface disease, follow up can be either with the patient's optometrist or your local general, corneal or oculoplastic clinic depending on severity and cause of the problem, as well as local protocols and guidelines.

PITFALLS

1. Recognition of acute dacryocystitis is important as failure to treat may result in orbital cellulitis or systemic complications. Acute dacryocystitis is almost always associated with nasolacrimal duct obstruction and in presence of an obstructed system, a DCR is recommended to prevent recurrence of infection.
2. Beware of a hard lump along the nasolacrimal sac, this maybe a tumour such as lymphoma or a squamous cell carcinoma.
3. Inflammatory diseases can also be a cause of nasolacrimal obstruction, though rare, but should the history suggest a systemic inflammatory disorder then further investigation is warranted via the oculoplastic clinic.
4. It is easy to be frustrated with patients attending eye casualty with what we sometimes consider a less important complaint, though it is prudent to remember that for the patient epiphora may be seriously damaging their quality of life and some simple reassurance can go a long way.

FURTHER READING

Sundaram V., A. Barsam, A. Alwitry, P. T. Khaw. *Training in Ophthalmology, the Essential Clinical Curriculum.* Oxford Specialty Training, 2016.

4   Trauma to the Eyelids and Periorbital Region

Abdus Samad Ansari

KEY POINTS

1. Consider mechanism and history: Blast injury, blunt trauma or metal on impact
2. Concurrent trauma should not be forgotten: Lid lacerations, penetrating periocular trauma
3. Look for suspicious findings: Peaked pupil, shallow anterior chamber or haemorrhagic chemosis
4. Always test and record visual acuity including the presence of a relative afferent pupillary defect
5. Be methodical in your examination and think anatomically from anterior to posterior and compare both eyes

DIAGRAM OF ALGORITHM

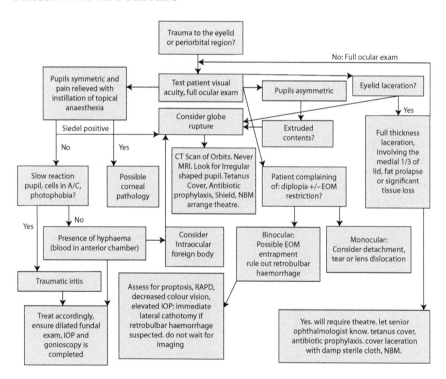

REFERRAL AND PRESENTATION

Trauma to the eyelids and periorbital region is not an uncommon cause of patient presentation to emergency departments throughout the United Kingdom. Traumatic insult to the periorbital region requires prompt assessment and intervention. Failure in the provision of optimal management in a timely manner may result in permanent visual loss. The vast majority of these patients are aged 18 to 45, with men demonstrating a fourfold greater risk of suffering from an eye injury compared to women. Despite the majority of these injuries being classified as minor; affecting the periorbital structures or the ocular surface, serious damage can be overlooked, especially in the instance of catastrophic or co-morbid trauma. To address this problem and optimise care in the setting of ocular trauma, a systematic and vigilant method of examination and intervention is required.

The type and extent of trauma is often linked to the mechanism of injury and history of presentation. The gravest injuries are those secondary to sharp entities, burns, as well as high velocity blunt and small objects. These can occur in any environment, be it at home, work or during recreational activities. Patients will usually present with a history of mechanical, chemical, and more rarely, radiation related trauma. Common presenting symptoms include that of acute onset reduction in vision, pain, epiphora, bleeding, and diplopia. It is essential that all traumatic injury patients undergo a complete physical survey to rule out any coexisting injury to the head or vital organs. You should not be afraid to ask for a complete skeletal survey (CT) by the referring physician, as this is not always the strength of the on call trainee ophthalmologist.

DIAGNOSIS

The effects of blunt trauma are likely to result in severe pain, blurred vision and epiphora. These patients have often sustained high velocity injuries to the eye and periorbital region. The cornea is frequently involved and it is thus important to assess for epithelial defects while also ruling out signs of oedema, abrasion and tears within Descemet's membrane. These patients may also present with limbal corneoscleral lacerations. Due to the nature of these injuries patients may additionally present with secondary hyphaema (blood located in the anterior chamber), which is often the result of damage to the structures located in the anterior or posterior chamber. Simply examining the pupil will reveal further evidence regarding the nature of structural damage caused by the injury; in particular it is important to look for signs of iridodialysis and lens stability.

Chemical and radiation burns should be suspected in patients presenting with conjunctival hyperaemia, chemosis and irritation to the periorbital region. Common signs include epithelial defects, corneal oedema, and inflammation within the anterior chamber; this can often cause secondary elevation of intraocular pressure. Radiation related injuries often present sub acutely within 6–12 hours post exposure.

The history will allow you to determine the potential site of injury and more importantly the likelihood of foreign body or ocular penetration. These patients often present with sharp pain, increased lacrimation, and a foreign body sensation with severe irritation. Although for the vast majority of these cases the clinician will be able to locate the culprit, it is nonetheless vital to rule out an intraocular foreign body (IOFB), especially with a history of explosion or when hammering and chiselling. Simple foreign bodies located within the ocular surface should be suspected when punctate epithelial erosions or linear vertical corneal abrasions are seen on the cornea. Quite often a subtarsal perpetrator is found embedded on lid eversion. When a conjunctival laceration is identified it is important to be suspicious of an injury affecting the deeper structures. Quite often this can mask an open globe injury and sometimes even an IOFB. The conjunctiva may appear to be

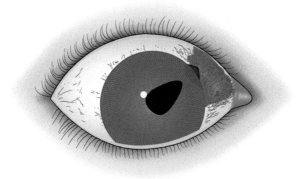

Figure 4.1   A peaked pupil indicative of an intraocular foreign body.

folded within itself with surrounding chemosis and subconjunctival haemorrhage. When confronted with these cases, the wound should be imaged and explored appropriately to ensure an accurate diagnosis to guide subsequent management. Signs that suggest an IOFB include an irregular shaped (peaked) pupil (see Figure 4.1), reduced IOP, vitreous haemorrhage, and intraocular inflammation. All structures of the eye should be examined systematically, with emphasis on the position and integrity of the lens and drainage angle.

By far the most daunting experience for any new trainee is the thought of managing an open globe injury. In the event of this serious injury, the appropriate identification, management and documentation are essential. These patients will often present with reduction in vision, severe pain and conjunctival haemorrhage. As mentioned earlier, the pupil can be a cardinal sign in confirming the diagnosis. This may be distorted and potentially prolapsing. The areas most likely to rupture include the limbus, the globe at the rectus muscle insertions and the cornea itself.

While the recognition of a lid laceration is often considered a simpler task in the ophthalmologic trauma survey, the loss of tissue can present substantial challenges to the assessing physician. Causes of lid lacerations can include dog bites, sheering forces when kicked and punched or direct sharp insult to the face. Lid lacerations are associated with symptoms of pain, lacrimation, periorbital oedema, and erythema. They can cause long term cosmetic issues and epiphora if not repaired well. Conversely, orbital wall fractures can present with acute onset diplopia, periocular ecchymosis, decreased sensation along the distribution of the infraorbital nerve and orbital emphysema.

CLINICAL EXAMINATION

Clinical examination should follow a systematic approach after assessing the general status of the patient. You should begin by simple bedside examination of the face, periorbital region and eyelids before finally examining the globe itself. It is vital that the patients' visual acuity for both eyes be recorded at initial presentation, as this is correlated to the final prognosis of injury and can also have medicolegal ramifications. Visual acuity may also be used to track the progression of recovery. Assess the patient's pupils and look for the presence of a RAPD, its shape, symmetry and both direct and consensual pupillary responses. The patient's ocular motility should be examined along with simple bedside confrontational fields.

A complete eye exam should be performed on all patients, with the form of test being usually guided by the location and mechanism of injury. Consider

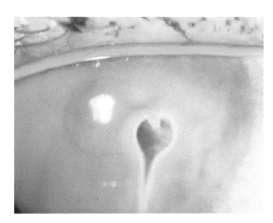

Figure 4.2 A Siedel positive test for investigating traumatic corneal injury. (Courtesy of Professor H S Dua, Consultant Ophthalmologist, Queens Medical Center, Nottingham, UK.)

retrobulbar haemorrhage in cases of blunt trauma in an eye with reduced optic nerve function, proptosis, reduced eye movements and severe pain. Saving vision is time dependent and sight saving canthotomy and cantholysis to reduce the orbital pressure should be performed now. The eyelids themselves should be examined for signs of trauma with particular attention being directed towards position of and size of any laceration, with the involvement of the lacrimal drainage apparatus being particularly important information. Involvement of the tarsal plate will always need formal repair, as will any damage to the eyelid margin, but if only skin is involved then steristrips may be used. If one or both canaliculi are involved it is important to be aware of this so that the oculoplastic team can plan their repair appropriately. A few simple sutures in eye casualty will not do; the vast majority of eyelid lacerations that are either full thickness or involve the lacrimal drainage network need formal repair in theatre. Adequate exploration of the wound can only be reliably undertaken in theatre, and a common pitfall is underestimating the depth or extent of lacerations in this area.

Slit lamp biomicroscopy will allow for accurate assessment of the ocular surface, lacrimal system, and integrity of the anterior globe. A Siedel test should be performed if a leak is suspected (see Figure 4.2). Dilated fundal examination should be completed on all patients with possible posterior segment involvement. Gonioscopy is useful in the detection of lesions such as angle recession in blunt trauma or to look for an IOFB located within the angle. However, this should not be performed in open globe injuries as the pressure may result in intraocular contents being squeezed through the wound. It is vital that the intraocular pressure is recorded; the form of tonometry will vary depending on availability and mobility of the patient. Lids should always be flipped to look for subtarsal foreign bodies.

Dilated fundal examination is useful to look for detachment, dialysis, tears, bleeds, commotio retinae or IOFB.

INVESTIGATIONS

Ocular/facial investigations should be considered on a case by case basis depending on the mechanism of injury and examination findings. First line imaging for traumatic ocular injuries should include a CT scan of the head and orbits. This is indicated if a foreign body or orbital wall fracture is suspected. This allows for complete evaluation of the integrity of the globe. Plain x-rays can also be used in the detection of an IOFB; however, the detection rate has been reported to be a low as 35%. Other imaging modalities to be considered include the use of B-scan ultrasound. This can be completed in a safe efficient manner and allows for quick evaluation of the posterior pole. This is not recommended in cases of suspected globe rupture due to the pressure involved. Although magnetic resonance imaging is contraindicated in cases of possible metallic IOFB, it can be useful in evaluating trauma, cranial injuries and retained wood materials. Ocular specific imaging to be considered include: optical coherence tomography, fluorescein angiography, and fundus autofluorescence. However, these are not commonly used in the acute phase of the disease, but could be used for photographic documentation.

Systemic laboratory tests to consider include routine blood tests and toxicology; particularly if you are planning on taking the patient to theatre. Patients with recurrent hyphaemas or of Afro-Caribbean descent who present with an acute hyphaema require an evaluation of sickle cell status. An ECG and medical work up may be required for patients undergoing general anaesthesia for the repair.

MANAGEMENT

The management of these conditions will vary depending on the form of injury sustained. Keep all patients nil by mouth if surgery is imminent.

Repair of eye lid lacerations can be repaired in the ED or by plastics or maxfax colleagues. However, in the case of dirty wounds, these should be washed out copiously and left open until sufficently cleaned. Lacerations involving the lid margins should be repaired with absorbable 6-0 and 5-0 vicryl sutures to bring the tarsal edges together again. Canalicular injuries will require oculoplastic repair usually under GA within the week to repair and preserve the lacrimal system. Whilst awaiting repair, ensure adequate corneal protection is provided when exposed.

Open globe injuries should not be explored until the patient is in theatre. The immediate care for the trainee is to ensure the eye is protected (covered with a clear plastic shield), and the patient is given systemic antibiotic and tetanus prophylaxis. The use of analgesia and antiemetics should also be considered. Principles of primary repair include: (1) the primary repairing the site of injury, (2) ensuring all leaking wounds are sealed, (3) treatment of contaminated vitreous with adequate intravitreal antibiotics, and (4) the removal of all anterior foreign bodies.

Injuries leading to epithelial loss at the level of the cornea or conjunctiva will usually require observation and topical antibiotic cream or ointment such as chloramphenicol is usually sufficient. Large, irregular conjunctival lacerations may require surgical repair, though this is not usually, and irregular abrasions.

Traumatic hyphaema secondary to blunt trauma often resolve with medical treatment which includes a tapering course of topical steroids, cycloplegia twice a day (i.e., cyclopentolate 1%) and close IOP monitoring. Treatment of traumatic anterior uveitis in the absence of a penetrating eye injury would involve a similar regime.

Fractures involving orbital bones do not usually require any acute management. These patients will require sub-acute surgical repair and orthoptic assessment including a HESS chart. This is usually coordinated between the maxillofacial team and ophthalmology. If however a retrobulbar haemorrhage is suspected, it is vital that a lateral cathotomy is completed. It is important that you check for increased IOP and central retinal artery perfusion. A lateral cathotomy is completed by releasing the lateral cathal tendon from the orbital rim and performing a catholysis (see Figure 4.3). This allows for a more anterior displacement of the globe, and thus a reduction in the intraorbital pressure as well as return of optic nerve and retinal circulation.

A table of the commonly used drugs when managing ocular trauma are summarised in Table 4.1.

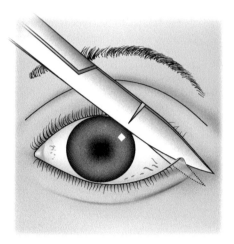

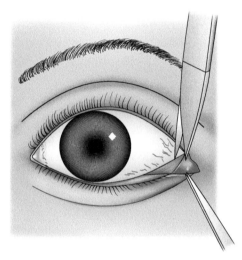

Figure 4.3   Performing a lateral canthotomy.

FOLLOW UP

The primary aims of follow up should include ocular surface protection, infection control, inflammation reduction and maintenance of normal intraocular pressure. Patients suffering traumatic ocular injury will require close and frequent monitoring. In particular, it is important to stay vigilant for any signs of endophthalmitis and retinal damage.

Patients that suffer from chemical or corneal epithelial defects require daily follow-up until improvement is documented. This is essential before treatment and visits can be tapered accordingly. This will of course vary depending on the severity and extent of damage caused by the exposure in question. Injuries that lead to the development of a hyphaema require daily follow up for the first 5 days due to the higher risk of re-bleeding during this period. Simple uncomplicated foreign bodies that are removed are unlikely to require follow up (unless located deep within the globe or orbit).

Table 4.1: Commonly Used Drugs Used in Managing Ocular Trauma

	Pharmacology	Mechanism of Action	Dosing	Contraindications	Side Effects
Chloremphenicol	Topical broad spectrum antibiotic often provided in the form of an ointment or cream	Bacteriostatic, works to inhibit protein synthesis works primarily on preventing protein chain elongation, inhibiting peptidyl transferase activity of bacterial ribosome	Application of 1 drop every 2 hours, reduce frequency as signs of infection are controlled	Acute porphyria	Bone marrow suppression, nausea, diarrhoea
Topical cycloplegia	Muscarinic receptor blockers including atropine, cyclopentolate, homatropine, scopolamine, and tropicamide	Muscarinic receptor block which works to dilate the eye (mydriatic) and prevent accommodation	One drop every 30 minutes for achieved effect	Children under three (should be avoided) acute glaucoma	Abdominal distension, arrhythmias, constipation, dizziness, dry mouth, flushing, headache, palpitation, psychotic disorder, vomiting, skin reaction

Deep lacerations and globe repairs must be monitored daily to ensure that wound leakage or secondary infection is identified early and treated in a timely manner. Secondary complications that may require further management include the development of glaucoma, cataract, and retinal tears, detachment or dialysis. Lid lacerations without globe involvement can be reviewed in 1–2 weeks, depending on a surgeon's surgical technique and planned suture removal.

PITFALLS

1. Common pitfalls include oversight of underlying ocular comorbidity. Thus, a thorough history, examination and recording of visual acuity are fundamental to the optimal care in acute ocular trauma.
2. Unfortunately, complications are not uncommon and clinicians should be aware of some of the consequences of medical error and oversight in the trauma setting; the most devastating of these being post-traumatic endophthalmitis. Patients will ordinarily present with marked inflammation, fibrin, hypopyon and intraocular inflammation. The most common microbial agents are that of coagulase-negative *Staphylococci* species and *B. cereus*. Treatment is a combination of systemic and intravitreal antibiotics; it is thus essential that prompt primary repair be completed alongside systemic antibiotics, if you wish to reduce the risk for complication.
3. Penetrating ocular injuries also have an estimated incidence of 0.2% of sympathetic ophthalmia. These patients can present anywhere from one week to years after the primary event. Signs can vary and can affect the posterior and anterior segment of the eye. It is vital that prompt aggressive therapy be initiated to preserve the vision once diagnosis is suspected.
4. Document, document, document—in the patient's notes, GP letter and by imaging. There are manifold medicolegal implications in these cases.

FURTHER READING

Blanch R. J., P. A. Good, P. Shah, J. R. B. Bishop, A. Logan, R. A. H. Scott. Visual outcomes after blunt ocular trauma. *Ophthalmology*. 2013; 120(8): 1588–1591. doi:10.1016/j.ophtha.2013.01.009.

Kuhn F. Ocular traumatology and the ocular trauma specialist. *Graefes Arch Clin Exp Ophthalmol* 2008; 246(2): 169–174.

Kuhn F., R. Morris, C. D. Witherspoon, K. Heimann, J. B. Jeffers, G. Treister. A standardized classification of ocular trauma. *Graefes Arch Clin Exp Ophthalmol*. 1996; 234(6): 399–403.

Romaniuk V. M. Ocular trauma and other catastrophes. *Emerg Med Clin North Am*. 2013; 31(2): 399–411.

Shankar P. V. Orbital trauma. In: R. Hoffmann Nunes et al. (eds.), *Critical Findings in Neuroradiology*. 2016. Springer, pp. 335–341.

Thylefors B. Epidemiological patterns of ocular trauma. *Aust N Z J Ophthalmol*. 1992; 20(2): 95–98.

5 Corneal Ulcers and Contact Lens Keratitis

Bushra Thajudeen

KEY POINTS

1. Corneal ulcers can be infective or non-infective.
2. Adequate history and careful examination of the anterior segment and adnexa are essential for managing patients correctly.
3. Corneal scraping from the ulcer edge should be performed before commencing treatment.
4. Tailoring the treatment according to host response is important in reducing toxicity.

DIAGRAM OF ALGORITHM

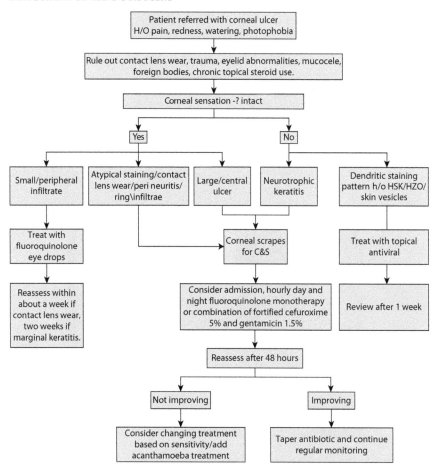

REFERRAL AND PRESENTATION

Corneal ulcers and contact lens keratitis constitute the majority of acute eye conditions presenting to the emergency clinic. Predisposing factors include trauma, corneal surgery, ocular surface disease, systemic diseases, immunosuppression and contact lens wear, which is the most common risk factor for infectious keratitis in developed countries.

Patients usually present with a red eye and symptoms of pain, photophobia, watering and visual disturbance, levels of which vary depending on cause and severity. Take a detailed history and remember to ask about associated symptoms such as discharge and itchiness as well as contact lens wear, past ocular history including surgery, as well as a medical history.

You may have to ask specifically for contact with chemicals, contact lens hygiene, previous herpetic infection, chronic dry eye and ocular surface problems. A systemic history should explore risk factors such as diabetic status, previous facial or brain surgery, rheumatoid arthritis, Sjögren's syndrome, systemic immunosuppression and malnutrition.

DIFFERENTIAL DIAGNOSIS

Adequate history and careful examination of the anterior segment of the eye is crucial, which will help identify if it is infectious or not and the risk factors or aetiology. Infectious corneal ulcers can be caused by bacteria, virus, fungi or acanthamoeba, and in some cases concurrent microbes may exist. Common non- infectious corneal ulcers include marginal keratitis, peripheral ulcerative keratitis (PUK), sterile corneal infiltrates associated with contact lens wear and toxic keratitis (contact lenses/solution or eye drops for example).

Marginal keratitis is caused by a hypersensitivity reaction against staphylococcal antigens in areas of lid margin and peripheral corneal contact. Symptoms include mild discomfort and redness in contrast for infective ulcers. Examination reveals evidence of chronic marginal blepharitis. Marginal infiltrates are separated from the limbus by a clear zone and the epithelial defect is usually smaller than the area of infiltrate (see Figure 5.1), which helps differentiate it from bacterial keratitis and PUK.

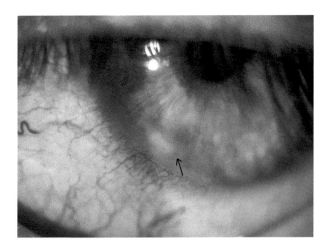

Figure 5.1 Marginal keratitis. (Courtesy of Professor H S Dua, Consultant Ophthalmologist, Queens Medical Center, Nottingham, UK.)

CLINICAL EXAMINATION

Clinical examination for corneal ulcers starts with the eyelids.

Eyelids: Assessment of eyelid position including looking for trichiasis, ectropion or entropion, floppy eyelids, inadequate lid closure and Bell's phenomenon are important. Look for all signs of blepharitis and associated features of meibomian gland dysfunction. Look for any evidence of a mucocoele which can be a risk factor for recurrent infections and is easily overlooked.

Conjunctiva: Look for foreign bodies (FB), scarring, large papillae, symblepharon or other earlier signs of cicatricial disease. Other findings, such as sutures and signs of previous eye surgery are also important. Remember to evert the eyelids and inspect for papillae, follicles, membranes or FB.

Cornea: Before staining the cornea make sure corneal sensation is assessed to rule out a neurotrophic cornea, as well as herpetic keratitis. Examination of the cornea should be systematic with careful assessment of the corneal epithelium, stroma and endothelium. Look for clues of underlying pathology in the other eye such as corneal dystrophies, corneal decompensation, immune conditions like peripheral ulcerative keratitis, Mooren's ulcer, ocular surface disease, toxic keratitis and so forth.

The ulcer: Measure and document the size and shape of the epithelial defect and infiltrate, noting the location, shape, depth, character of infiltrate margin (suppurative, necrotic, feathery, soft, crystalline), and colour of the corneal ulcer. Assess the depth and extend of stromal infiltrate. Look for anterior chamber reaction which can vary from a few cells to hypopyon. Severe anterior chamber reaction is characteristic of suppurative infective keratitis.

Fluorescein staining: Gives additional information, such as the presence of dendrites, pseudo dendrites, loose or exposed sutures, epithelial defects, or pre-existing ocular surface disease. The corneal staining pattern will itself give a clue to the aetiology. If you get a dendritic pattern of epithelial staining, it's most probably herpetic keratitis. If you see localised corneal epithelial punctate staining, with no other significant findings except for some epithelial irregularity in a symptomatic contact lens wearer, always consider acanthamoeba keratitis and look closely for perineural infiltrates. Also, corneal staining helps in assessing the response to treatment. If the epithelial defect is getting smaller than before and lesser in size than the infiltrate, it is an indication of adequate response to treatment.

Documentation: Clinical signs need to be accurately noted as it helps when monitoring response to treatment. Measure the size of epithelial defect and infiltrate and document it along with other signs including height of the hypopyon, blood vessels, immune ring, perineuritis with a clearly drawn and labelled illustration. The size of the epithelial defect will obviously change after corneal scrape, so consider taking photographs prior to performing a corneal scrape.

INVESTIGATIONS

Although the clinical picture can give clues to the aetiology, it is important to obtain corneal scrapes for microbiology before commencing treatment.

Corneal scrapes and swabs: Any ulcer that is central, large, deep, chronic or atypical should be scraped. A #15 Bard-Parker blade or a large gauge needle or kimura spatula can be used to obtain a large enough tissue sample from the advancing borders of the infected area. Remove all necrotic tissue from the ulcer before scraping as this is full of dead useless stuff. Samples should be sent for gram stain and culture for bacteria and fungi. If there is any suspicion of acanthamoeba, samples should be obtained for separate special staining and culture depending on local methods. Remove fluorescein dye from the eye prior to using swabs to improve test accuracy.

Corneal biopsy: Is useful if the ulcer is resistant to treatment and cultures have been negative. Biopsy samples should be sent for microbiology and pathology examination. This will, however, never be undertaken in eye casualty as an initial investigation.

Confocal microscopy: Is used to look for trophozoites and cysts of acanthamoeba and fungal hyphae. It is best performed before corneal scrape for a clearer image for accurate interpretation.

Contact lens and case: It is also a good idea to culture the contact lenses/cases in contact lens wearers; however, the majority will grow acanthamoeba anyway. If anything, looking at the condition of the contact lens case can provide clues as to the likelihood of such infection.

DIAGNOSIS

Bacterial ulcers: Gram positive bacteria characteristically cause well circumscribed ulcers. Staphylococcus aureus usually causes round or oval lesions with dense infiltration and a distinct border. Streptococci cause acute and highly suppurative ulcers which can be associated with a sterile hypopyon. Gram negative bacteria cause soupy infiltrates that are not well defined and associated with copious mucopurulent discharge. Rapid progression, dense stromal infiltrate, liquefactive necrosis and corneal perforation are the characteristics of pseudomonas infection. *Gonococcal* ulcers are associated with hyper purulent conjunctivitis and chemosis and can rapidly result in corneal perforation (see Figure 5.2).

Viral keratitis: Common viral pathogens include: herpes, varacella-zoster and adenovirus. The main corneal manifestations of herpes simplex infection include infectious epithelial keratitis, neurotrophic keratopathy, necrotizing stromal keratitis, immune stromal keratitis, and endothelitis. Herpes simplex keratitis is characterised by dendritic epithelial staining pattern with terminal bulbs (see Figure 5.3). Associated skin lesions and previous history can give a clue towards aetiology. Herpes zoster keratitis is characterized by dendritic lesions which are smaller and finer than herpes simplex dendrites and have tapered ends without terminal bulbs, commonly called pseudo-dendrites. A skin rash respecting the

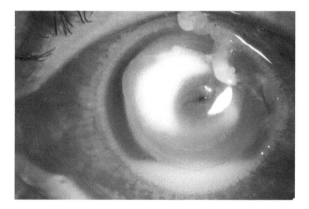

Figure 5.2 Typical pseudomonas keratitis with corneal melt. (Courtesy of Professor H S Dua, Consultant Ophthalmologist, Queens Medical Center, Nottingham, UK.)

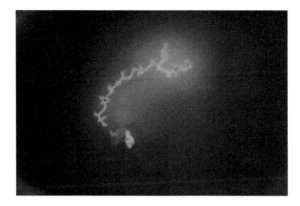

Figure 5.3 Dendritic ulcer. (Courtesy of Amy-lee Shirodkar, Specialist Registrar, University Hospital of Wales, Cardiff, UK.)

midline helps in distinguishing shingles from HSV infection. In both cases, corneal sensation will be reduced. In disciform keratitis there will be stromal infiltrate, localised corneal oedema and keratic precipitates on the underlying endothelium (see Figure 5.4). Healing epithelial defects, varicella-zoster pseudo dendrites and acanthamoeba are often misdiagnosed as HSV dendritic ulcers.

Adenoviral keratitis is associated with a recent upper respiratory tract infection with conjunctivitis, and presents with 'adeno-spots' – subepithelial deposits with pinpoint staining. This is a condition commonly picked up by eye casualty doctors.

Acanthamoeba keratitis: Symptoms disproportionate to the clinical signs is characteristic of acanthamoeba keratitis due to irritation of the corneal nerves and hence usually missed in the early assessment. There will be history of contact lens wear with poor hygiene or contact with water. Clinical signs can be very subtle with irregular corneal surface and punctate staining. Acanthamoeba can also present as a dendritic staining pattern, and hence one should always rule out acanthamoeba keratitis when a contact lens wearer presents with a dendritic ulcer. Gradual enlargement and coalescence of the infiltrates lead to a ring infiltrate and stromal infiltrate can lead to corneal melt. Perineural infiltrates are pathognomonic and

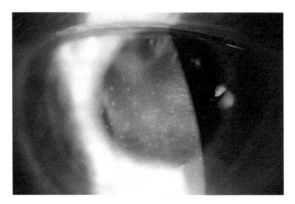

Figure 5.4 Disciform keratitis. (Courtesy of Professor H S Dua, Consultant Ophthalmologist, Queens Medical Center, Nottingham, UK.)

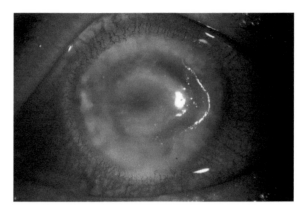

Figure 5.5 Acanthamoeba keratitis. (Courtesy of Professor H S Dua, Consultant Ophthalmologist, Queens Medical Center, Nottingham, UK.)

are visible as white lines corresponding to inflammation of the corneal nerves (see Figure 5.5). Acanthamoeba related ulcers can be differentiated from HSV because they are raised, rather than ulcerated, and do not necessarily stain with fluorescein.

Fungal keratitis: Uncommon in temperate countries, the predisposing factors include systemic immunosuppression or long-term use of topical steroids, with fungal ulcers being seen most commonly following corneal injuries with vegetative matter. Yeasts like candida cause a yellow-white densely suppurative infiltrate while filamentous fungi like *Aspergillus* and *Fusarium* cause yellow-white stromal infiltrate with fluffy margins, feathery extensions and satellite lesions. They can also be associated with hypopyon which contain the fungal hyphae.

MANAGEMENT

General principles: The majority of bacterial keratitis with small infiltrates or peripheral location can be managed with empiric therapy using commercial, broad-spectrum topical antibiotics. Central or large corneal infiltrates extending to the deep stroma need corneal scraping for microbiological culture and specific topical antibiotic therapy. Hospital admission should be considered if the patients are unlikely to comply with treatment, especially intensive treatment in the initial few days. Later, if the ulcer becomes resistant to treatment, we must consider stopping all therapy and re-scraping the ulcer to look for any other organism. Some cases will benefit from use of amniotic membrane to enhance healing. In cases with progressive keratitis or impending perforation, a tectonic or therapeutic penetrating keratoplasty may be needed. Promotion of epithelial healing is important for a non-healing sterile ulcer and can be improved by debridement of necrotic corneal stroma, lubrication, and/or temporary tarsorrhaphy.

Antibiotics: Topical antibiotic eye drops achieve high levels of tissue concentration and are the preferred choice for infective ulcers. Ointments may be used especially overnight in less severe cases but may impair the penetration of co-administered drops. Systemic antibiotics may be considered in severe cases with scleral or intraocular extension of infection or impending perforation.

Cycloplegics: Help with pain relief. Debriding the corneal epithelium also helps in better penetration of antibiotics and decreasing the bacterial load, so worry not too much about how much epithelium comes off during scraping.

Oculosurface protection: Surgical techniques such as temporary tarsorrhaphy will help with healing when ulcers are neurotropic, chronic or caused by corneal exposure due to poor lid closure.

Toxicity: Drug toxicity due to prolonged use or unsuitable type of medication can cause increasing discomfort, redness, discharge and persistent epithelial defect despite eradication of infection.

Steroids: Can be started once there are signs of clinical improvement as they reduce inflammation, improve comfort and minimize the corneal scarring. However their timing and use is still unclear and some argue that it can worsen the ulcer by promoting bacterial and fungal growth and there is no clear evidence that it improves the final visual outcome.

SPECIFIC TREATMENT

Bacterial keratitis: Empirical treatment with fluoroquinolone eye drops or combination of fortified cefuroxime 5% and gentamicin 1.5% should be started after obtaining corneal samples, depending on local protocols. The drops should be used half hourly or hourly for the first 48 hours during the day and night before reassessing the ulcer for response to treatment by reassessing the VA, size of the infiltrate, ED and AC activity. Treatment can also be tailored to microbiology results.

Fortified antibiotics are not commercially available and are prepared by your local pharmacy and have a short shelf life. Monotherapy with fluoroquinolones (third or fourth generation) alone are just as effective as combination therapy with fortified antibiotics. For large ulcers with dense infiltrates, intensive treatment in the initial period is crucial.

Viral keratitis: Herpetic epithelial keratitis responds to aciclovir 3% ointment or ganciclovir 0.15% gel, each administered 5 times daily for 7–10 days. Oral antiviral therapy is indicated in immunodeficient patients and may also be effective alternatives to topical treatment when the latter is poorly tolerated, or in resistant cases. Some centres advocate swab confirmation and debridement. Almost certainly avoid topical steroids.

Disciform keratitis: Initial treatment is with topical steroids with oral antiviral cover. Topical steroid treatment should be deferred if there is an epithelial defect; patients should be started on antiviral treatment first and once the epithelium has healed with intensive lubricants, steroids can then be commenced.

Herpes zoster ophthalmicus: Treat with oral aciclovir for 7–10 days. Topical antivirals are needed only if the cornea is involved.

Acanthamoeba keratitis: If there is some doubt about whether the causative organism is bacterial or protozoal it is much safer to treat as for acanthamoeba than the reverse. Intensive treatment depending on clinical suspicion and local protocols with either:

- Polyhexamethylene biguanide (PHMB) 0.02% with either hexamidine 0.1% or propamidine 0.1% (Brolene®)

or

- Chlorhexidine digluconate (0.02%) and hexamidine 0.1% or propamidine 0.1% (Brolene®)

Topical treatment should be hourly day and night for 48 hours before review. Some may combine a fluoroquinolone whilst awaiting microbial/confocal confirmation. Topical steroids should be avoided in the immediate stage. Again debridement of epithelium helps drug penetration. Early involvement by the corneal service is recommended. Relapses are common as treatment is tapered, and it is therefore necessary to continue treatment for many months.

Fungal keratitis: For filamentous fungi, natamycin is effective while yeasts like candida respond better to amphotericin and azoles including itraconazole or voriconazole. Because most antifungals are only fungistatic, treatment should be continued for at least 12 weeks. A broad-spectrum antibiotic should also be considered to address or prevent bacterial co-infection. Systemic antifungals may be considered if there is severe infection with threatened perforation, endophthalmitis, or the patient is immunocompromised.

FOLLOW UP

After the initial 48 hours of intensive drops, treatment must be tailored to the host response. Signs of clinical improvement include improving visual acuity, decreasing pain, reduced amount of discharge, re-epithelialization, sharper demarcation of margins, decreasing density and size of the infiltrate, reduced corneal oedema and anterior chamber reaction.

Intense topical antimicrobial treatments can be toxic to the cornea, hence it is important to start tapering drops if there are early signs of improvement and clinical stability, such as closure of an epithelial defect.

If no improvement is evident following 48 hours of intensive treatment, the antimicrobial regimen should be reviewed, including contacting the microbiology laboratory to obtain the latest report.

There is no need to change the initial therapy if this has induced a favourable response, even if cultures show a resistant or additional organism.

PITFALLS

1. Treating a dendritic ulcer in a contact lens wearer as herpes simplex instead of acanthamoeba.
2. Failure to recognise and treat local risk factors like abnormalities of eyelids/eyelashes, mucocele, dry eye and so forth.
3. Not checking the corneal sensation is another pitfall as it could delay diagnosis.
4. Failure to obtain corneal scrapes before starting treatment might save time in the short term but cause a whole host of problems should the patient not respond to treatment. In this eventuality a period of washout by withdrawing treatment to re-scrape may be needed. Always chase the results before starting steroids.
5. Over treating leading to toxic epitheliopathy is another pitfall as it results in non-healing chronic epithelial defects, which is common with prolonged and frequent topical aciclovir use in particular.

FURTHER READING

Denniston A., P. Murray. *Oxford Handbook of Ophthalmology*, Oxford University Press, 2014.

Mannis M. J., E. J. Holland. *Cornea.* 4th edition, Elsevier, 2016.

Weisenthal R. W. Basic and clinical science course, Section 8: External disease and cornea, American Academy of Ophthalmology, 2019–2020.

6   Corneal Defects, Abrasions and Foreign Bodies

Magdalena Popiela

KEY POINTS

1. Corneal abrasions are superficial losses of corneal epithelium, which heal quickly. They usually occur as result of mechanical trauma, so don't forget to look for other signs of blunt or penetrating eye injury.
2. Fluorescein 2% is useful in diagnosis as it stains the epithelial defect.
3. Corneal foreign bodies should be removed to allow for epithelial healing to occur. Don't forget to look for multiple foreign bodies, signs of penetrating eye injury and to evert the lids.
4. Topical antibiotics are used to prevent subsequent bacterial infection in cases of corneal abrasions and post corneal foreign body removal.

DIAGRAM OF ALGORITHM

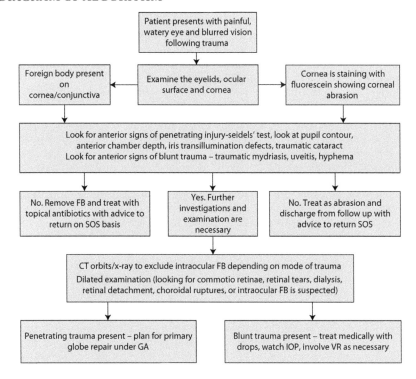

REFERRAL AND PRESENTATION

In the presence of normal corneal sensation, corneal defects and foreign bodies will be extremely painful. Patients will present with a sore, watery eye and variable amounts of blurred vision. Presentation of both corneal defects and corneal foreign bodies is usually acute, and as the epithelium heals symptoms will improve.

Corneal epithelial defects (ED) and corneal foreign bodies (FB) occur as a result of mechanical trauma and need to be examined for in this context, including everting the eyelids. Corneal defects can also be iatrogenic as a result of several surgical procedures: post corneal crosslinking, post laser refractive surgery or superficial keratectomy. In these cases debridement of the epithelium is performed purposefully but also, not uncommonly, can occur iatrogenically after intravitreal injection or cataract surgery – when one mistakenly scratches the eye with a piece of equipment.

In cases of mechanical trauma the mode of injury needs to be elicited from the history, remembering that high impact injuries carry a risk of penetrating globe damage. Abrasions are a one off event but the initial trauma (especially fingertip or sharp paper cut injuries) can lead to recurrent erosions, a syndrome whereby recurrent abrasions occur due to irregularity of healed epithelium and weakened adherence to its basement membrane. Recurrent corneal erosion syndrome can present many years after the initial trauma. Recurrent erosions occasionally occur in the presence of a corneal dystrophy, where irregularity of the epithelium, due to abnormal deposits in the cornea, are to blame. Patients usually experience intense pain, foreign body sensation and photophobia on waking, as the weak corneal epithelium is torn off as the eyelid opens up, having adhered to it as the cornea naturally dries overnight.

In cases of retained foreign bodies, certain materials can cause a greater inflammatory reaction than others. Inflammation on the cornea appears as a grey infiltrate around the foreign object. Wood, copper, iron and steel have the highest inflammatory reaction potential. Nickle, zinc and aluminium are pro-inflammatory. Glass, lead, plastic and porcelain are inert and any injury with vegetative material will carry the risk of fungal infections.

DIFFERENTIAL DIAGNOSIS

The cornea is made up of different layers: epithelium, Bowman's layer, stroma with pre-Descemet's layer, Descemet's membrane and endothelium (see Figure 6.1). Corneal defects are synonymous with abrasions and involve focal losses of epithelium. The regenerative power of the corneal epithelium is extraordinary; it heals quickly and usually without scarring. However corneal healing is largely dependent on a healthy corneal nerve plexus and an adequate amount of limbal epithelial stem cells. The cornea is one of the most densely innervated parts of human body, with corneal nerves originating from the trigeminal nerve ganglion. Central epithelial nerve plexuses can contain as many as 600 nerve terminals/mm^2, acting as afferent sensory nociceptors transducing mechanical, thermal and chemical stimuli as well as sensation of pain. Corneal nerves serve an important function in maintenance of corneal health and play vital role in epithelial healing. Any condition which affects the trigeminal nerve leads to delayed healing and subsequently can lead to loss of corneal transparency.

Corneal defects: Can be seen in dry eyes, corneal ulcers (viral, bacterial, fungal and parasitic), corneal exposure due to lid or lash malposition, chemical or thermal burns, recurrent erosion syndrome due to corneal dystrophies, in the presence of limbal stem cell deficiency or in cases of neurotrophic corneas.

Superficial epithelial defects: Need to be distinguished from epithelial defects associated with underlying corneal thinning, present in active peripheral ulcerative keratitis or necrotizing stromal keratitis.

Penetrating globe injuries: Need to be considered, especially when triaging, in setting of trauma for both corneal abrasions and corneal foreign bodies.

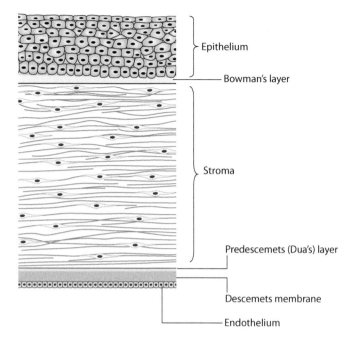

Epithelium

Bowman's layer

Stroma

Predescemets (Dua's) layer

Descemets membrane

Endothelium

Figure 6.1 The layers of the cornea.

CLINICAL EXAMINATION

Examination might be difficult as patients will be in pain. Instillation of topical anaesthesia at the start will make patients more comfortable and allow easier and more comprehensive anterior segment examination and measurement of VA. However, check corneal sensation beforehand where indicated.

Corneal abrasions: Are best seen with blue light after instillation of fluorescein dye, which will stain cornea denuded of epithelium and defects will glow green (see Figure 6.2).

Corneal FB: Are usually immediately visible on anterior segment examination. Don't forget to examine the eye for multiple foreign bodies, especially those hiding under the upper lid. In the presence of linear corneal epithelial defects, the upper lid must be everted, as this is a sign of repetitive scratching on blinking. In practice, however, it is better to evert the lids of every single patient presenting with an epithelial defect and a red eye.

Ocular examination: Because both corneal abrasions and corneal FBs are caused by ocular trauma, further examination needs to be tailored to the history and presence of anterior segment signs suggestive of more substantial damage to the eye. These include the presence of pigment on the conjunctiva, positive Seidel's fluorescein test, flattening of anterior chamber, irregularity/peaking of the pupil, iris transillumination defects and presence of traumatic cataract.

In cases of blunt trauma anterior uveitis, hyphaema and traumatic mydriasis might be present in conjunction with a corneal defect. Perform dilated examination for patients with these signs. In cases of penetrating injury where the iris is plugging the corneal wound and imaging shows no intraocular foreign body, dilated examination can wait until after primary globe repair is performed. In these cases undilated fundal examination should be attempted.

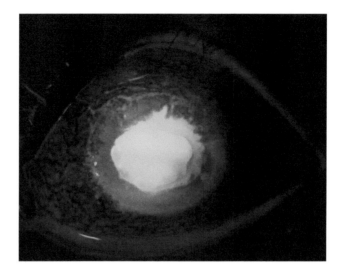

Figure 6.2 An epithelial defect highlighted by using a blue filter after fluorescein installation.

INVESTIGATIONS

Investigations are not necessary in cases with clean epithelial defects that are not associated with any underlying conditions or penetrating injury. Superficial corneal foreign bodies with no signs of penetrating eye injury also do not need to be investigated further.

Ocular imaging: Should be used to photograph severe trauma and anterior segment OCT used for baseline corneal thickness measurement in cases of corneal thinning.

Imaging: Facial x-ray or CT with orbital views needs to be performed if penetrating eye injury or intraocular foreign body are suspected.

DIAGNOSIS

The diagnosis is clinical and greatly aided by the use of fluorescein and blue light for epithelial defects (see Figure 6.2). Corneal or conjunctival foreign bodies will be immediately visible on clinical examination without the use of fluorescein dye. Other corneal defects include: dellen, desmatoceles, melts and perforation.

MANAGEMENT

Epithelial defects: Will heal spontaneously in the presence of a healthy tear film, limbal stem cells and normal corneal sensation. It is customary to treat epithelial abrasions with topical antibiotics to prevent secondary infections, usually with chloramphenicol 4 times per day for one week, but many will improve with lubricants alone. In the case of contact lens wearers with an epithelial defect, treat with topical fluoroquinolones one drop 4–6 times per day for one week to provide cover against *Pseudomonas*. Patients should be advised not to wear their contact lenses while the cornea heals.

Debride: If the epithelium is irregular around the defect it should be debrided to aid healing. Use of lubricating eye drops also promotes epithelial healing and helps to alleviate discomfort. In cases of corneal abrasions acquired through sharp cut trauma, it might be beneficial to continue long term lubricating drops and ointment to reduce the risk of recurrent erosion syndrome occurring at a later date.

Bandage contact lenses: Should be reserved for the treatment of 'clean' epithelial defects, which do not carry the additional risk of acquired infections. Bandage contact lenses can be considered in recurrent erosions and post-operatively in iatrogenic abrasions as a means of controlling the pain and aiding healing. Topical antibiotics should be used to prevent secondary infection, and ointment preparations should be avoided. If it is planned to leave the lens in the eye for longer than a week then preservative free drops should be used.

Antibiotic ointment and double padding: Of the eye can also be an effective strategy to deal with corneal erosions as it might help to alleviate symptoms of pain; although this approach is best avoided in cases with high risk of secondary infection, whereby a pair of tinted glasses may help.

Pain relief: Various topical treatments have been advocated for pain management, though the evidence for their effectiveness is not robust. Dilating drops like cyclopentolate or atropine relax the ciliary muscle and are thought to ease ciliary muscle spasm, which contributes to symptoms of pain. Topical non-steroidal anti-inflammatory drugs are another option to consider. The use of topical anaesthetic drops generally is avoided, as this can delay healing and promote infection with prolonged and frequent use. The use of topical anaesthetics is the accepted routine treatment strategy for patients with corneal defects post corneal surgery. Warn patients that each of the above treatments will cause stinging on drop application and that dilating drops cause blurred vision and an enlarged pupil.

Foreign bodies: Corneal or conjunctival foreign bodies need to be removed as they prevent the epithelium from healing and are risk factors for infective keratitis. If, however, the FB is chemically inert and becomes incorporated in the corneal tissue with corneal epithelium healing over the top of it, and the patient maintains good vision, then just observe it.

Removal of a corneal foreign body: After local anaesthetic drops, a wet sterile cotton bud can be initially used to try and dislodge the foreign body. If this is unsuccessful a green needle (or smaller) can be used to remove the foreign body, using a scooping movement. Be mindful of the young male patient who may be prone to fainting on you. Similarly, a rust ring can be debrided either with a needle or Alger brush if available. If the rust ring is deep or difficult to remove, try repeating the procedure a few days later after ointment use.

Topical treatment: Following removal of the foreign body, treatment includes topical antibiotics, usually Chloramphenicol in drop or ointment form, 4 times per day for a week. Patients should be advised to wear protective glasses in the future to prevent repeated injury, especially if it was acquired within the workplace.

FOLLOW UP
Discharge: For traumatic corneal abrasions or corneal foreign bodies in the presence of no other worrisome features no follow up is necessary. Corneal abrasions will heal without a scar in the majority of patients, but can occur if foreign bodies penetrate deeper within the cornea due to the non-healing nature of corneal basement membranes. But these scars will fade with time.

Patients should be warned to return if symptoms don't improve within a few days. Pain is the first symptom to improve, whereas blurred vision can take longer to settle. Patients with foreign bodies, especially if removed from central cornea, might experience some degree of visual loss. Usually it is mild, however these patients can be referred to designated corneal clinics for visual rehabilitation if necessary.

Children with abrasions: Special consideration is given to children, where follow up is arranged 2–5 days after the initial injury for a visual acuity check and further examination, when pain is no longer an issue. Always be mindful of safeguarding issues.

Contact lens wearers: Follow up should also be considered for contact lens wearers and patients attaining injury with vegetative matter, since these groups are at higher risk of subsequent infective keratitis. If a bandage contact lens is used in management of a corneal abrasion it needs to be removed, so arrange follow up for these cases as appropriate (usually within 5–7 days for simple abrasions, or longer if lens is planned to be left in the eye, in cases of recurrent erosion syndrome). If recurrent erosion is a frequent issue then refer to the corneal team for definitive management, to save the patient having to re-attend eye casualty a thousand times for the same painful problem.

Post-op corneal patients: Any patient with a corneal graft should be referred urgently in the presence of an epithelial defect or damage to the graft or laser flaps.

PITFALLS AND HOW TO AVOID THEM

1. Don't forget to exclude penetrating globe injuries and look for other signs of blunt trauma. Take a good history and perform a tailored examination, ask about pupil shape and peaking when triaging/taking referral.
2. Don't forget to look for multiple foreign bodies, especially ones hiding under the top lid.
3. Don't forget that deep rust rings can be removed a few days after the initial attempt to allow for some healing, making subsequent debridement more superficial and easier.
4. Don't forget to look at the other eye. In cases of recurrent erosion syndrome the other asymptomatic eye might show signs of a corneal dystrophy.
5. Don't forget to examine the lids and lashes. Their abnormal position might delay healing but might also point to another aetiology for the corneal defect. The presence of blepharitis and/or meibomian gland disease with multiple small punctate erosions over the inferior cornea is suggestive of dry eyes. Early corneal exposure can show the same signs of inferior punctate staining before the epithelial defects get bigger.
6. Don't forget to consider early infective keratitis as a differential diagnosis of epithelial defects especially in the presence of risk factors such as contact lens wear, long-term topical steroid use, previous corneal graft surgery, ocular surface disease and previous herpetic eye disease history.
7. Don't forget to check corneal sensation in corneal defects which have not healed within two weeks of presentation. These are then treated as neurotrophic ulcers and require specialist input. These epithelial defects might have raised and whitish edges. Patients will also not experience the same degree of pain as patients with normal corneal sensation.

FURTHER READING

External Disease and Cornea. *Basic and Clinical Science Course, Section 8.* San Francisco: American Academy of Ophthalmology, 2017–2018.

Maguire J. I., A. P. Murchison, E. A. Jaeger. *Wills Eye Institute 5-Minute Ophthalmology Consult.* Lippincott Williams & Wilkins, 2012.

Pandey J. Ocular foreign bodies: A review. *Clin Exp Ophthalmol.* 2017.

7 Photophobia and Anterior Uveitis

Gwyn Samuel Williams

KEY POINTS

1. There are many different causes of photophobia
2. Iritis and anterior uveitis are synonyms
3. Always dilate patients with anterior uveitis to examine the fundus
4. Only some cases of anterior uveitis need further investigation

DIAGRAM OF ALGORITHM

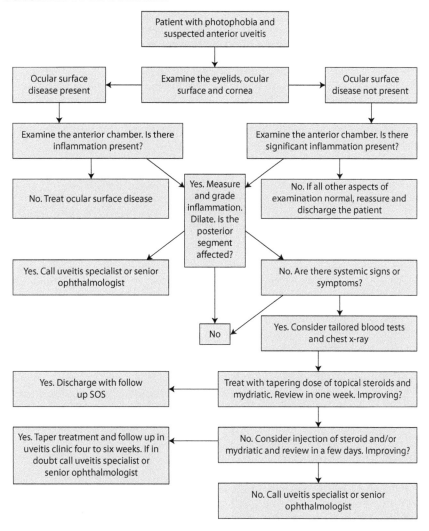

REFERRAL AND PRESENTATION

Photophobia implies a painful sensitivity to light, nothing more, nothing less. Some health professionals seem to automatically link photophobia with iritis, more properly termed anterior uveitis, but there are in fact several other important causes that need to be excluded before such a diagnosis can be made. Patients with sudden onset acute light sensitivity, particularly if this is the first ever episode, may present to accident and emergency. This is usually not so convenient as after a 4-hour wait the harried casualty officer usually has not much more ophthalmic experience than their week's worth of training in medical school. After using a broken down slit lamp to ascertain that, yes, the patient is photophobic will then call the on call ophthalmologist without a visual acuity test and without having performed a useful examination.

More helpfully, a patient may attend an optometrist such as those affiliated in Wales with the Welsh Eye Care Scheme (WECS) who are trained to perform a proper ocular examination and who will then ring up the on call officer with useful information and a good stab at a diagnosis. England has a similar scheme termed the Minor Eye Condition Service (MECS), and the Scottish have their own too. Patients presenting to their general practitioner with such symptoms will sometimes, but not always, tell a story whereby they were given a tube of chloramphenicol for their 'conjunctivitis' and sent away.

Iritis and anterior uveitis are synonymous, and by their very nature, are recurrent. So after a few flare ups patients learn the best way to access hospital eye care, which is usually slightly different in every hospital in the land. So if a patient calls up with 'another flare up of iritis', they are usually right about this and pointless excursions to accident and emergency or community optometrists in such circumstances are best avoided, unless your system is inflexible.

DIFFERENTIAL DIAGNOSIS

Photophobia implies an anterior segment pathology, when related to ocular pathology. Whilst anterior uveitis, inflammation of the iris, is indeed the condition that classically causes this symptom, there are others to be aware of as well. Inflammation of the cornea of whatever aetiology, a contact lens related ulcer, a marginal keratitis or keratitis of any cause for that matter, can all cause photophobia. Likewise tear film instability, dry eyes, blepharitis and indeed conjunctivitis can also cause photophobia, though usually of a lesser magnitude than anterior uveitis itself. Raised pressure in the eye in the form of closed angle glaucoma does not usually cause photophobia as the patient is commonly more concerned with vomiting into a sick bowl to be much bothered at someone shining a light in their eye.

Migraine also famously causes photophobia as do other neurological conditions, but it is unusual for such patients to present to eye casualty as a possible iritis due to the accompanying headache and recurrent nature of the condition prompting most sufferers to seek the solace of a dark room.

Anterior uveitis can be categorised based on time between occurrences, duration and presence of a granulomatous inflammation. Sarcoidosis for example is more likely in what is termed a 'granulomatous' anterior uveitis: inflammation with large greasy so called 'mutton fat' KPs in the presence of iris nodules.

CLINICAL EXAMINATION

Visual acuity should be documented accurately, and the patient then examined at the slit lamp. The cornea should be examined for signs of keratitis and ulceration, with fluorescein then instilled to highlight any punctate epithelial erosions, dendritic ulcers, abrasions or any other epithelial pathology.

The eyelids: Are examined for meibomian gland dysfunction and blepharitis, which mainly involves looking for scales at the level of the eyelashes or rows of blocked meibomian glands behind the eyelashes, which can sometimes secrete a toothpaste-like substance when handled.

Anterior chamber: Once these other causes for photophobia are excluded, you can then examine the anterior chamber proper. Obviously if a patient is a known uveitic, possibly HLA B27 positive, and the attack feels like a 'typical flare up' then these stages may be hurried, though it is unwise to skip altogether a look at other structures lest something be missed, such as a dendritic ulcer, for example.

The reason anterior uveitis causes such pronounced photophobia is that the iris constricts to light, and if it is inflamed, as with trying to flex a broken leg, the movement causes pain. This is also why pupil dilation can be such a relief for patients, as it is the equivalent of a leg splint for the eye. It is useful to bear this in mind when examining such patients and reducing the width and strength of the slit lamp beam is a kindness.

Cells and flare: Are what are measured when examining patients with suspected iritis. Aqueous flare is proteinaceous leakage from anterior segment blood vessels. The four hallmarks of inflammation are calor (heat) rubor (redness) dolor (pain) and tumor (swelling), and with inflammation of the iris the rubor manifests as what is termed 'ciliary injection' where the redness of the affected eye is much more pronounced immediately behind the limbus. The tumor, or swelling, manifests as protein leaking into the anterior chamber, and it is this that constitutes the flare. It is graded as in Table 7.1, based on how clearly defined the details of the iris are. Grade 4 flare appears like a solid lump of fibrin with a yellowy hue that can block utterly the view of the fundus and fill much of the anterior chamber.

Cells are measured by reducing your slit lamp beam to a 1 mm by 1 mm segment, increasing the illumination and magnification as much as possible and focusing on the anterior chamber in front of the pupil after directing the light beam in from an angle of around 30 degrees. Cells appear as small motes of dust as in your living room suspended in a sunbeam on a bright spring day. As with dust, the cells can be seen to lazily pass in and out of the beam of light depending on the natural convection currents in the anterior chamber. The grade of severity of the cells present is dependent on their number and is as described in Table 7.2. Grading cells and flare is vital so that improvement or deterioration can be measured in subsequent visits. This system was agreed to internationally by the Standard Uveitis Nomenclature (SUN) working group in order to standardise uveitis care.

The presence of a hypopyon indicates severe inflammation and in these cases endophthalmitis must always be ruled out.

Table 7.1: How to Grade Flare According to the Standard Uveitis Nomenclature (SUN) Working Group Classification

Degree of Blur Looking at the Iris	Flare Grading
None	–
Hardly any	+
Definite blur but iris details still clear	++
Obvious blur with iris details hazy	+++
Fibrinous flare/plastic aqueous	++++

Table 7.2: How to Grade Cells According to the Standard Uveitis Nomenclature (SUN) Working Group Classification

Number of Cells Observed in 1 mm by 1 mm Beam	Cell Grading
0	–
1–5	+/–
6–15	+
16–25	++
26–50	+++
>50	++++

Keratic precipitates (KPs): Are small accretions of inflammatory debris that collect on the posterior aspect of the endothelium, and due to gravity and convection currents are inferiorly located. If the KPs are smaller and evenly distributed this is called a 'stellate' distribution and implies Fuchs heterochromic iridocyclitis, a condition which as the name suggests also has a differently (usually lighter) coloured iris in the affected eye. It is important to make this distinction as Fuchs does not require treatment for the inflammation as the cells will never clear completely and rather review in a dedicated uveitis clinic is warranted. Figure 7.1 illustrates the difference between KP distributions in these two conditions.

Iris: Whilst looking at the iris sometimes granulomata, or nodules, are apparent. These are focally thickened rounded areas of iris which if located at the pupillary margin are termed 'Koeppe nodules' and if located elsewhere 'Busacca nodules'.

Measure IOP: Uveitis can be associated with increased intraocular pressure so Goldmann tonometry is essential. There is a variant of anterior uveitis called Posner–Schlossman syndrome that typically presents with mild inflammation and very high pressures in the affected eye.

Dilate: Uveitis if only anteriorly located is also termed iritis but before this can be determined for sure, the fundus needs to be examined, and for this to be done adequately, the patient MUST be dilated. Always, always dilate anterior uveitis patients to examine the fundus. If the fundus is normal, a posterior element to the uveitis can be ruled out but if there are retinal changes then senior help must be summoned. Anterior uveitis can also cause cystoid macular oedema, which can be picked up on optical coherence tomography scanning. One of the commonest reasons uveitis specialists are sued is because a patient with anterior uveitis was not dilated, and an important blinding posterior pathology, usually acute retinal necrosis, was missed.

INVESTIGATIONS

Less is definitely more when it comes to investigating anterior uveitis in the casualty room. If the signs and symptoms are typical and the patient young, Caucasian and otherwise systemically well, there is not usually any need to perform any investigations.

Bloods: Absolutely under no circumstances go wild on the blood form and tick every box as false positive results can be very misleading. ANA is a particularly

(a)

(b)

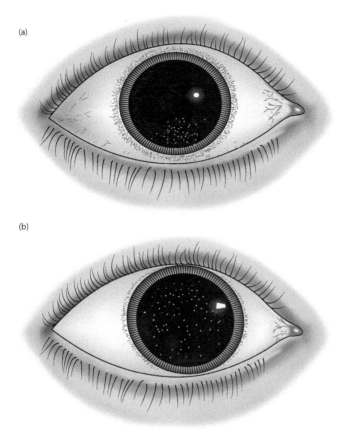

Figure 7.1 Keratic precipitate distribution in (a) normal anterior uveitis and (b) Fuchs heterochromic iridocyclitis.

useless test in these circumstances and lupus should be so far down the list of differential diagnoses that it is best forgotten, at least in eye casualty.

If the patient has had multiple episodes, it is customary to perform a HLA B27 blood test, regardless of the suspicion of ankylosing spondylitis, though this does not alter prognosis but can give patients some peace of mind that there is a 'cause' to their troubles and it can help them adjust their lives accordingly. If there are systemic symptoms such as respiratory, joint or skin issues in addition to the uveitis then a CRP, ESR, ACE, FBC, U and E and a chest x-ray may be indicated.

Very occasionally a masquerade syndrome will be the cause of the uveitis and under these circumstances it is almost always best for this to be investigated by the uveitis specialist. Your job as casualty officer is to recognise an atypical case and refer on appropriately.

DIAGNOSIS

The diagnosis of anterior uveitis is a clinical one but should systemic conditions such as sarcoidosis or tuberculosis be suspected then additional testing is required.

From an emergency ophthalmology perspective only order those blood tests mentioned above, and only then if needed, plus a chest x-ray again if circumstances dictate.

Asking about systemic symptoms and past medical history is vital in helping you select which, if any, blood tests are ordered. Patients with uveitis after recent eye surgery should have endophthalmitis on your list of differentials, while patients that have had a trabeculectomy at any time presenting with uveitis should be considered to have endophthalmitis until proven otherwise. Beware the white bleb in a red eye.

MANAGEMENT

Photophobia: In general pain will ease with treatment of the underlying cause. However, in the interim, cycloplegia, dark glasses, topical NSAIDs and oral analgesia may give some relief.

Anterior uveitis: Is treated with topical steroids in a tapering regime, usually consisting of maxidex or predforte hourly for a week, every other hour for a week, qds for a week, tds for a week, bd for a week and od for a week. Cyclopentolate 1% bd is usually given for the first week to prevent posterior synechiae formation and to reduce pain and photophobia in the initial severe period. The patient should be reassessed sooner in cases with poor fundal view but the majority in 1–2 weeks in eye casualty or clinic to assess for improvement, always keeping careful watch over the intraocular pressure and inflammation levels. Again, always examine the posterior segment at each visit with dilated fundoscopy. Should the patient be responding positively to treatment then continue the regime and discharge from the hospital eye service with instructions to contact the department again should there be any problem is the usual procedure.

Should the patient not be improved at one week then injecting 1 mL of subconjunctival betnesol (4 mg) after topical anaesthesia can help things along. Similarly should the pupil still be stuck down with posterior synechiae at one week then 0.5 mL of subconjunctival mydricaine may do the trick. Of course, both can be combined and delivered as one injection if needed at the same time. Later, should the patient still not respond, then referral to a uveitis clinic or senior ophthalmologist is needed. Patients should NOT be seen repeatedly in eye casualty with non-responding uveitis time and time again as valuable time will be lost in preventing permanent damage to vision.

FOLLOW UP

Discharge: Should the patient be improving at follow up then discharge is warranted with an emergency phone number to get back in touch in the event of any difficulty arising, depending on local policy.

Follow up: Should this not be the case, then injection as highlighted above and follow up in a further week, or few days, is warranted but should the patient still not be responding to treatment then referral to a specialist is indicated.

Recurrent AAU: Patients with known recurrent anterior uveitis flare ups do not need to be reviewed after a week if their disease course is usually predictable and they know their own condition well. If any systemic condition is suspected at the first visit, or any major complicating factor or unusual presentation, then immediate referral to a uveitis specialist or senior ophthalmologist may be needed.

PITFALLS

1. The biggest pitfall is not dilating a patient with anterior uveitis for a look at the fundus. It might be that it is all anterior, but if there is a posterior element that is missed for want of dilation then this may be a blinding experience for the patient and a career damaging event for the ophthalmologist. ALWAYS DILATE PATIENTS WITH ANTERIOR UVEITIS.
2. Failure to properly examine the ocular surface is another pitfall. Corneal ulcers can cause cells to appear in the anterior chamber and adding intense topical steroid to a corneal ulcer may not necessarily be in the patient's best interest.
3. Following non-responding patients up in eye casualty for too long, possibly by passing them on to different ophthalmologists who have never seen them before, is bad medicine. Likewise failing to measure the intraocular pressure is negligent.
4. Lastly in some eye departments there seems to be a culture of labelling normal eyes 'iritis' without having seen a single solitary cell on the basis that it may be very mild. It is a reasonable postulation that the real reason for this is that it is much simpler to hand over a bottle of steroid drops than to have a difficult conversation about having not found a cause for the patient's symptoms. Either way, this should be avoided for obvious reasons.

FURTHER READING

Williams G. S., M. Westcott. *Practical Uveitis: Understanding the Grape.* Taylor & Francis Group, 2017.

8 Red Eyes after Cataract Surgery and Other Operations

Annie See Wah Tung

KEY POINTS

1. Endophthalmitis must always be considered a differential in post-operative uveitis
2. Have a low threshold in reviewing post-operative patients in the emergency clinic
3. Pain and reduced vision are red flags when accompanied with post-operative red eyes
4. If symptoms are significant but unexplained, arrange early review and 'safety net' with warning signs

DIAGRAM OF ALGORITHM

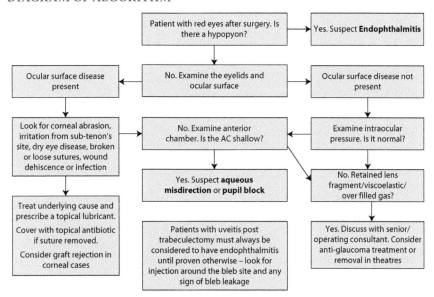

Patient with red eyes after surgery. Is there a hypopyon? → Yes. Suspect **Endophthalmitis**

No. Examine the eyelids and ocular surface

Ocular surface disease present ← → Ocular surface disease not present

Look for corneal abrasion, irritation from sub-tenon's site, dry eye disease, broken or loose sutures, wound dehiscence or infection

No. Examine anterior chamber. Is the AC shallow?

Examine intraocular pressure. Is it normal?

Treat underlying cause and prescribe a topical lubricant. Cover with topical antibiotic if suture removed. Consider graft rejection in corneal cases

Yes. Suspect **aqueous misdirection** or **pupil block**

No. Retained lens fragment/viscoelastic/over filled gas?

Patients with uveitis post trabeculectomy must always be considered to have endophthalmitis until proven otherwise – look for injection around the bleb site and any sign of bleb leakage

Yes. Discuss with senior/operating consultant. Consider anti-glaucoma treatment or removal in theatres

REFERRAL AND PRESENTATION

Post-operative cataract surgery patients are abundant due to the frequency of the procedure all over the country, and it is not uncommon for them get a red eye despite our best efforts, lest eye casualty get inundated by calls from the worried well. Most experienced surgeons would warn their patients about a little subconj bleeding and redness. If however the patient also experiences irritation, photophobia, watery or sticky eyes, they will start to worry something might be wrong, and correctly so, as post-operative, they should be warned to look out for these signs and symptoms.

If the patient calls you via the emergency ophthalmology phone line detailed on their leaflet, obtain a brief history, including the type of operation they had, the surgeon's name and as much information as possible about the problem itself, such as the speed of onset and the severity of symptoms over the course of the post-operative period. Sometimes all they need is reassurance, and this may be in form of telephone advice or a clinic consultation.

The role of a casualty ophthalmologist is to detect sight-threatening disease such as post-operative endophthalmitis or raised intraocular pressure. Early management in these cases can significantly alter prognosis, and therefore clinicians should be vigilant. Generally, these sight threatening conditions are accompanied with pain; however, this should not be relied upon, as the pain and visual disturbance of a corneal abrasion alone can be quite severe. Patients may complain of reduction in vision if they had good pre-operative vision. If you work in a unit that is referral based, my advice is to have a low threshold to see post-operative patients urgently when referred. If you work in a walk in centre, ensure good post-operative patient education is conveyed to prevent non-urgent cases, such as subconjunctival haemorrhage (SCH) presenting in the early hours of the morning (if at all).

DIFFERENTIAL DIAGNOSIS

Below is a list of potential post-operative complications that can lead to a red eye.
Infective:

- Acute post-operative endophthalmitis
- Blebitis
- Conjunctivitis

Suture/injection site trauma:

- Pyogenic granuloma
- Suture granuloma
- Conjunctival laceration from sub-tenon injection
- Sub-conjunctival haemorrhage
- Eyelid wound dehiscence
- Retrobulbar haemorrhage

Inflammatory:

- Post-operative uveitis
- Scleritis

Pressure related:

- Retained viscoelastic
- Wound leak with hypotony
- Steroid response

Ocular surface:

- Dry eyes (Povidone iodine, exposure, reduced blinking due to anaesthetics)
- Corneal abrasion (from speculum or instruments)
- Allergy (Povidone iodine/ post-operative drops/preservatives/suture material/tape)

CLINICAL EXAMINATION

History: Prior to examination, you need to establish whether the patient is on anti-coagulants, anti-platelets or has pre-existing bleeding disorders, which puts them at a higher risk of SCH. You would also want to know if they are at higher risk of severe inflammation due to a history of uveitis. Was the operation routine or complicated? What was the mode of anaesthesia? Check if the patient is diabetic or immunocompromised as this increases their risk of infection.

Examination: Visual acuity must be checked and documented at each post-operative review. On the slit-lamp, examine the patient for any risk factors of ocular surface disease such as blepharitis, mucocoele, entropion or ectropion. Lid swelling and inflammation are also signs associated with endophthalmitis. Is there any yellow discharge from the eye? Perform a conjunctival swab of any discharge prior to examining the ocular surface specifically looking at wound and injection sites. If the patient complains of discomfort with blinking or eye movement this is more likely to be due to an ocular surface problem. Use fluorescein 2% to check for a wound leak from corneal incisions, sutures, trabeculectomy and vitrectomy port sites. In post-filtration surgery in glaucoma cases, look for any signs of pus-discharge, a milky bleb and wound leak suggestive of blebitis. In post-corneal graft patients, look for loose sutures that may be a source of irritation or infection and signs of graft failure or rejection. Look for signs of recurrent corneal disease in those with previous herpetic disease.

Anterior chamber (AC) assessment: Post-operative inflammation in the AC is expected generally in the first 4 weeks following intraocular surgery. Pay attention to any signs of flare, hypopyon, fibrin or vitreous prolapse. Vitreous can be directly visualised as strands in the AC, peeking of the pupil margin or as a wick at the wound. Also assess the AC depth. If shallow and associated with a high IOP, suspect aqueous misdirection, pupil block or a suprachoroidal haemorrhage. If the AC is deep with a high IOP, this may be due to retained viscoelastic, an over-filled eye with gas from VR cases or tight sutures/wound hydration as well as inflammation and a multitude of other less common causes. Toxic Anterior Segment Syndrome (TASS) is a severe post-operative complication presenting a few hours after intraocular surgery resulting from drug or exotoxin toxicity. This is an inflammatory condition.

Posterior segment: Always attempt to perform dilated fundoscopy, or B-scan in cases of post-operative corneal oedema significant enough to block the view of the posterior segment. Determine whether there are vitreous cells or debris present. The presence of vitreous inflammation with anterior chamber inflammation is strongly suggestive of endophthalmitis. A B-scan is important in identifying signs of retinal detachment, choroidal effusion or supra-choroidal haemorrhage, especially in eyes with no direct view. Indirect biomicroscopy with a 20D or 28D lens gives a better view in a gas filled eye.

INVESTIGATIONS

Endophthalmitis: If acute post-operative endophthalmitis is suspected, perform ultrasound B-scan to assess extent of vitritis and retinal involvement. Perform AC tap and vitreous biopsy with injection of intravitreal antibiotics as soon as possible, as per local protocol. Samples should be sent to microbiology for culture and sensitivity, and PCR performed if possible.

Blebitis: Swab the conjunctiva around the bleb for culture and sensitivity. Consider AC tap depending on extent of intraocular involvement. Bleb-associated endophthalmitis (BAE) is investigated and treated as per post-cataract endophthalmitis.

DIAGNOSIS

Post-operative ocular surface disease: Is a diagnosis based on clinical assessment.

Post-operative infection: It may be difficult to distinguish between severe post-operative inflammation and post-operative infection. When there is significant intraocular inflammation, it should be managed as suspected endophthalmitis. Microbiology helps with confirming the diagnosis of an infective cause.

Common organisms:

- Acute endophthalmitis (1–7 days): *Staphylococcus epidermidis, Staphylococcus aureus* and *Streptococcus* spp
- Chronic endophthalmitis (>1 week-months): *Propionobaceterium acnes, Staph. epidermidis,* fungi
- Early BAE: coagulase-negative *Staphylococcus*
- Late BAE: *Streptococci* spp

Post-operative raised intraocular pressure (post-trabeculectomy, cataracts or corneal graft):

With shallow AC:

- Pupillary block (central AC deeper than periphery)
- Aqueous misdirection (shallow central and periphery)
- Supra-choroidal haemorrhage (shallow central and periphery)

With deep AC:

- Tight sutures/flap
- Internal block (iris, ciliary body, blood clot)
- Flat bleb/Tenon's cyst

MANAGEMENT

Ocular surface disease:

- Remove underlying cause of irritation (where appropriate)
- Changing to preservative free drops
- Topical lubrication +/− steroids
- Oral NSAIDs/steroids for diffuse anterior sclerotic changes

Corneal graft patients:

- Bleb leak or wound leak, consider bandage contact lens (with preservative free antibiotic cover) or re-suturing
- Increase antibiotic/steroid cover if corneal suture removed to prevent infection or rejection

- Discuss with corneal surgeon early if continuous sutures are used as likely to require re-suturing

Post-operative blebitis:

- Hourly fortified topical antibiotic: vancomycin 50 mg/mL, amikacin 20 mg/mL or ceftazidime 100 mg/mL

- Oral antibiotics: Fluoroquinolone e.g. moxifloxacin 400 mg OD or ciprofloxacin 750 mg BD

- Consider admitting patient for close monitoring

- Any signs of significant reduced vision or vitritis, treat as endophthalmitis

Post-operative endophthalmitis:

- Consider admission to ward

- Intravitreal biopsy and injection of antibiotics (vancomycin 1 mg/0.1 mL for gram positive cover, AND ceftazidime 2 mg/0.1 mL or amikacin 0.4 mg/0.1 mL for gram negative cover)

- If vision is PL at presentation, early vitrectomy is found to be beneficial, discuss with VR

- Use of intravitreal steroid (dexamethasone 0.4 mL/0.1 mL) is controversial but may reduce sequelae of inflammation

Post-operative raised intraocular pressure (post trabeculectomy, cataracts or corneal graft):

With shallow AC:

- Pupillary block – miotics, peripheral iridotomy/iridectomy

- Aqueous misdirection – strong cycloplegic, aqueous suppressant, disrupt vitreous face (laser posterior capsulotomy/hyaloidotomy, needle aspiration, pars plana vitrectomy)

- Supra-choroidal haemorrhage – manage IOP, wait for clot to lyse, drain with sclerotomy

With deep AC:

- Tight sutures/flap – digital pressure, releasable sutures/laser suture lysis

- Internal block (iris, ciliary body, blood clot) – gonioscopy to look for obstruction

- Flat bleb/Tenon's cyst – subconjunctival injection of 5-FU/MMC, bleb needling

FOLLOW UP

Always inform the operating surgeon and consultant as soon as possible to discuss further management. Most trabeculectomy and corneal graft patients are reviewed frequently by the operating team in the immediate post-operative period for complications of surgery. This should be undertaken in the specialist clinic and not eye casualty.

Ocular surface disease: If no other red flag signs are present and a clear cause for the red eye is identified, treat the underlying cause and follow your post-operative plan and treatment regime.

Post-operative infection: Patients should be admitted for frequent review. If no/poor response to treatment is observed after 48 hours, consider repeating the intravitreal antibiotics +/− vitreous biopsy under the guidance of the consultant in charge.

Post-operative raised intraocular pressure: Follow up, depending on cause, within two days to recheck IOP, and refer to the operating team or glaucoma service for further follow up.

PITFALLS

1. *Anterior segment ischaemia (ASI):* is an uncommon but serious complication usually following squint surgery involving three or more muscles. ASI occurs due to disruption to the blood supply from the anterior ciliary arteries. It has also been reported in patients after retinal detachment with scleral buckling or encirclement due to compromise of blood vessels. Patients in this group are usually older and have predisposing atherosclerosis or possibly haemoglobinopathies. Early signs of ASI include cells and flare in the anterior chamber which may resemble post-op inflammation. Other signs may include corneal oedema, hypotony, irregular pupil and rubeosis. In advanced cases, it may cause necrosis of the anterior segment and phthisis bulbi. Treatment is with topical or systemic steroids to suppress inflammation and topical cycloplegics to prevent synechiae.

2. It is easy to dismiss patients with a red eye or discomfort assuming it is part of the normal post-operative course. The duty of care to our patients continues after the operation and post-operative management forms an important part of the patient's overall surgical experience. With trabeculectomy and corneal surgery, post-operative care is also vital to surgical success. Infective complications can progress rapidly and often lead to poor prognosis. Therefore, have a low threshold in reviewing post-operative patients in the emergency clinic.

FURTHER READING

Denniston A., P. Murray. *Oxford Handbook of Ophthalmology*, Oxford University Press, 2014.

Forster R. K. The endophthalmitis vitrectomy study. *Arch Ophthalmol.* 113(12): 1995; 1555–1557.

Guidelines on the management of cataracts in adults. NICE Guidelines 26 Oct 2017.

Lee J. P., J. M. Oliver. Anterior segment ischaemia. *Eye* 4: 1990; 1–6.

Apparent Sudden Visual Loss: An Essential Approach

Colm McAlinden

KEY POINTS

1. Always consider giant cell arteritis as a cause of visual loss
2. Measure blood pressure in cases of suspected papilloedema
3. Always consider acanthamoeba keratitis in contact lens users

DIAGRAM OF ALGORITHM

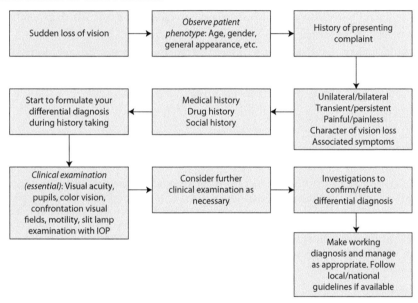

REFERRAL AND PRESENTATION

Sudden loss of vision is an ophthalmic emergency and patients should be seen without delay. Patients are likely to be very worried and typically present directly to hospital (emergency department or eye department) or attend a community optometry practice. Occasionally patients may present to their general practitioner or are referred by another medical team within the hospital.

As with everything in medicine, the history is key. One must ascertain if the sudden loss of vision is unilateral or bilateral, transient or persistent, painful or painless, the nature of the vision loss (complete loss with no light perception, cloudy, blurred, distorted, partial or shadow), and associated symptoms (red eye or headache). Patients may complain of total loss of vision, i.e. black out like someone switched off the lights, very murky vision – like looking through a dirty fish tank or looking through fog.

DIFFERENTIAL DIAGNOSIS

Whilst observing the patient phenotype during history taking, it is important to start formulating the differential diagnosis to ensure the pertinent questions are asked. Below is a non-exhaustive list of the main causes of sudden loss of vision, distinguished by transient and persistent causes:

- *Transient:* amaurosis fugax, papilloedema, migraine, impending central retinal vein occlusion, ischaemic optic neuropathy, ocular ischaemic syndrome, intermittent angle closure, vertebrobasilar insufficiency, sudden change in blood pressure, optic nerve head drusen and orbital lesions (may have vision loss on eye movement). Duration of loss can vary from a few seconds to a few hours depending on the cause.

- *Persistent:* central retinal artery or vein occlusion, ischaemic optic neuropathy, giant cell arteritis, vitreous haemorrhage, retinal detachment, optic neuritis, corneal disease (including hydrops), acute glaucoma, trauma, orbital cellulitis, endophthalmitis, neovascular age-related macular degeneration, and lens dislocation.

Functional vision loss is also a differential that may coexist with organic disease. Purely functional vision loss is not a diagnosis of exclusion but rather, must be supported by positive findings on examination that demonstrate normal visual function (see Chapter 25 for further reading).

CLINICAL EXAMINATION

The examination will be focused dependent on the history and differential diagnosis. However, it is important to conduct a comprehensive clinical examination as often there is discordance between symptoms and signs.

Optic nerve function: Visual acuity (VA) is a useful starting point to procure an understanding of the severity of vision loss. This can be followed with further assessment of optic nerve function such as pupil responses with a specific emphasis on the presence or absence of a relative afferent pupillary defect (RAPD), colour vision (if possible in view of vision loss; usually possible with Ishihara plates with a VA $\geq 6/18$) and confrontation visual fields (formal automated static perimetry can be arranged for more detailed assessment).

Ocular examination: Ocular motility at this point may elicit any co-existing incomitancy or pain on eye movement (associated with optic neuritis). Slit lamp examination will enable an examination of the anterior and posterior segments including intraocular pressure (IOP) measurement.

Other: In cases of suspected giant cell arteritis, palpate the superficial temporal artery pulses; an absent pulse and thickened vessel is highly suspicious of giant cell arteritis. This is best palpated just anterior and superior to the tragus (above the zygomatic arch of the temporal bone). In cases of suspected central nervous system disease (e.g. stroke, multiple sclerosis), it may be necessary to perform a neurological examination (cranial nerve examination and upper and lower limb neurological examination). In cases of amaurosis fugax, central retinal artery occlusion and ocular ischaemic syndrome, it can be useful to auscultate the carotids for bruits.

INVESTIGATIONS

Investigations should be used to confirm or refute the diagnosis. In some cases such as central retinal artery occlusion (CRAO) presenting within 90 minutes or so, you should commence treatment and save the investigations for later.

Ischaemic events: Such as amaurosis fugax and CRAO require further investigation. It would be worthwhile to ask colleagues what local pathways or protocols exist for the management of these patients, as it often differs among hospitals. Typically, basic investigations are ordered by the ophthalmologist including blood tests and a carotid ultrasound Doppler, with the patient being followed up by a physician (e.g. stroke team) for further investigations and management or in a fast-track transient ischaemic attack (TIA) clinic.

GCA: Although giant cell arteritis is most commonly associated with anterior ischaemic optic neuropathy, it must be considered in any potentially ischaemic ocular event including CRAO and posterior ischaemic optic neuropathy. The triad of blood tests including erythrocyte sedimentation rate (ESR), C-reactive protein (CRP) and platelet count should be sent to the lab and marked as urgent. Rarer conditions such as ocular ischaemic syndrome require more detailed investigations.

Papilloedema: Is exclusively bilateral disc swelling secondary to elevated intracranial pressure which prompts neuro-imaging and onward referral to the necessary specialty dependent on cause. Blood pressure should also be measured before jumping to expensive imaging to ensure the papilloedema is not secondary to malignant hypertension. As an ophthalmologist, one will be asked frequently to check for papilloedema by medical or optometric colleagues. Although not exclusively, the presence of spontaneous venous pulsation suggests there is unlikely to be raised intracranial pressure. Formal static perimetry can be useful to assess blind spot enlargement or constricted fields.

Ultrasonography (known as a B-scan [brightness-scan]) can be helpful in differentiating disc oedema and disc drusen, as the latter may appear reflective (see Figure 9.1). Fundus autofluorescence and fundus fluorescein angiography (FFA) can also be useful adjuncts. Optical coherence tomography (OCT) is a non-invasive imaging modality providing a cross-section of the retina. This can be performed centred on the disc and one can assess if a 'lazy V' pattern of the subretinal

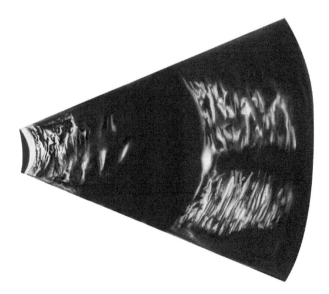

Figure 9.1   A B-scan image demonstrating optic disc drusen.

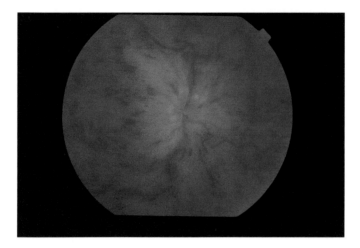

Figure 9.2 Fundus picture of a patient with a central retinal vein occlusion. (Courtesy of Miss Susmita Bala, Consultant Ophthalmologist, Queens Medical Center, Nottingham, UK.)

hyporeflective space (more in keeping with papilloedema) or a 'lumpy bumpy' pattern (more in keeping with disc drusen) is evident (see paper by Johnson et al. *Arch Ophthalmol.* 2009, for further reading – reference below).

Retinal vein occlusion: Is a common eye disease, usually presenting in the elderly (see Figure 9.2). Patients should have their blood pressure measured, blood tests for diabetes, full blood count (FBC) and ESR. Routine thrombophilia testing is not usually recommended in retinal vein occlusions but certain features in the history and patient age may warrant further investigation via the haematologist.

Optic neuritis: In typical cases of optic neuritis (age 20–50, unilateral, worsening over hours or days, recovery starts within 2 weeks, retrobulbar pain, reduced colour vision and an RAPD) further investigations may not be necessary. In atypical cases, it would be judicious to investigate further for possible progressive optic neuropathy.

Exogenous endophthalmitis: Is an emergency whereby every minute matters. Local procedures should be followed but typically anterior chamber tap and vitreous biopsy (followed by intravitreal antibiotics) is performed (see Chapter 8 for further reading).

OCULAR IMAGING

B-scan: In cases of no fundal view, whatever the cause, it is imperative to perform B-scan ultrasonography to assess the integrity of the retina. This is a skill that all ophthalmologists in training should acquire. A vitreous haemorrhage for example will appear as a mobile reflective vitreous opacity (see Chapter 11 for further reading).

OCT: An OCT scan will enable the detection of retinal thickening with retinal cysts and sub-retinal fluid. OCT imaging is also used to monitor the effects of treatments. In cases of neovascular age-related macular degeneration, FFA and OCT are also important investigations in the diagnosis and management of the disease (see Chapter 12 for further reading).

FFA: is a useful investigation to help categorise ischaemic and non-ischaemic vascular compromise, predicting the visual outcome, assessing the risk of neovascularisation and guiding treatment. It is important to check for contraindications to FFA such as renal impairment and an allergy to fluorescein.

DIAGNOSIS

Careful history and examination should narrow the differential diagnosis substantially. Further investigations as per the differential diagnosis should, in most cases, provide the diagnosis. As with any diagnosis, it should be deemed a working diagnosis and open to challenge. Dealing with uncertainty is part and parcel of medicine, but in situations of high uncertainty, one should have a low threshold to seek opinion or advice from senior or specialist colleagues and always rule out GCA. This really cannot be emphasised enough.

MANAGEMENT

Triage time dependent emergencies as a priority.

Central retinal artery occlusion: Causes inner retinal hypoxia leading to acute coagulative necrosis followed by complete loss of the nerve fibre layer, ganglion cell layer and inner plexiform layer. Typically there is a significant delay in the presentation of the patient to the ophthalmologist. If the patient is seen within 24 hours of the loss of vision, it is common practice, although limited evidence of benefit, to rapidly reduce intraocular pressure (IOP) (e.g. 500 mg of intravenous acetazolamide, ocular massage, anterior chamber paracentesis – see Figure 9.3). As mentioned above, one of the key tasks is to consider and investigate for giant cell arteritis. Not considering this and if left untreated, it may lead to an ischaemic event in the contralateral eye. Giant cell arteritis is treated with high dose corticosteroids. All patients with central retinal artery occlusion should have a cardiovascular work-up and onward referral to a stroke team or TIA clinic.

Papilloedema: The main role of the ophthalmologist is to diagnose the presence of papilloedema and record the optic nerve function. Physicians in training seem to

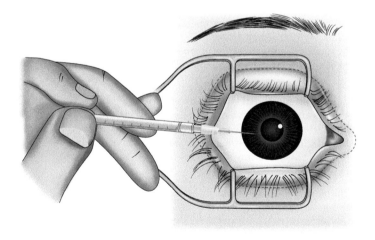

Figure 9.3   Performing an anterior chamber paracentesis.

have lost the skill of ophthalmoscopy. Patients are managed by instigating neuro-imaging and referring on to the appropriate medical team (see Chapter 21 for further reading).

Vitreous haemorrhage: The management of vitreous haemorrhage will largely depend on the underlying cause and duration. In cases of known proliferative diabetic retinopathy with previous pan retinal photocoagulation and a flat retina on B-scanning, it may be appropriate to observe for spontaneous recovery. In cases without diabetic retinopathy, one must have a high suspicion for a retinal tear and discuss/refer onward to the vitreoretinal (VR) service as urgent surgery may be required. See Chapter 16 for further reading.

Optic neuritis: The decision whether to treat with corticosteroids remains controversial. Intravenous corticosteroids may speed visual recovery but does not appear to affect the final VA recovery. Whilst oral steroids are unhelpful (follow local protocols and refer to neurology).

Retinal vein occlusion: Management depends on a range of factors including whether it is central, branch or hemiretinal, ischaemic or non-ischaemic, presence or absence of neovascularisation, anterior chamber angle open or closed, IOP, VA and features on FFA. Treatments for macular oedema include anti-vascular endothelial growth factor (VEGF) therapy, dexamethasone implant (Ozurdex® from Allergan) and laser. The Royal College of Ophthalmologists has produced guidelines on the management of retinal vein occlusions considering all these specific factors. Neovascular age-related macular degeneration is usually managed by a dedicated macular service with anti-VEGF therapies including ranibizumb (Lucentis® from Novaritis) and aflibercept (Eylea® from Bayer). Ultimately, refer patients to your MR service for definitive management, remembering that neovascular complications should either be seen by them within 2 weeks and if this is not guaranteed consider performing pan retinal photocoagulation in clinic.

Exogenous endophthalmitis (post-operative): Is an emergency whereby every minute matters. Local procedures should be followed but typically, anterior chamber tap and vitreous biopsy (followed by intravitreal antibiotics) is performed (see Chapter 8 for further reading).

FOLLOW UP

CRAO: Although the prognosis for visual improvement in cases of central retinal artery occlusion is extremely poor, patients should be monitored in clinic for the development of ischaemia and resulting neovascularisation. Iris neovascularisation can lead to neovascular glaucoma resulting in a painful blind eye.

Papilloedema: Patients with papilloedema, with a common cause being idiopathic intracranial hypertension (IIH), are typically followed up by the ophthalmologist for visual fields and optic nerve assessment. These findings along with symptoms are used to titrate dosing in the treatment (e.g. acetazolamide) of IIH by neurology or general medicine. It must be stressed that the term 'papilloedema' is specifically reserved for optic disc swelling secondary to raised intraocular pressure and never any other cause.

Retinal vein occlusion: Cases need to be closely monitored, whether this is in a dedicated macular service whilst the patient is receiving anti-VEGF therapy for macular oedema or in an outpatient clinic. Apart from monitoring the effects of treatment, it is important to observe for secondary complications including neovascularisation.

AMD: Patients with neovascular age-related macular degeneration are typically followed up in a macular service with intervals depending on the treatment regime (e.g. fixed dosing or treat and extend).

Optic neuritis: Typical cases of optic neuritis should be followed up in clinic to monitor visual recovery and in cases of non-recovery, the consideration for alternative causes of optic neuropathy.

PITFALLS

1. One of the biggest pitfalls is not considering giant cell arteritis in an age appropriate case of visual disturbance or loss, including central retinal artery occlusion.
2. In cases of optic disc swelling, always measure blood pressure to exclude malignant hypertension.
3. Always consider acanthamoeba keratitis in contact lens related microbial keratitis, especially if the symptoms of pain outweigh the clinical signs.

FURTHER READING

Bagheri N., B. N. Wajda. *The Wills Eye Manual: Office and Emergency Room Diagnosis and Treatment of Eye Disease;* 6th ed. Wolters Kluwer, 2017.

Bowlings B. *Kanski's Clinical Ophthalmology – A Systematic Approach.* 8th ed. Elsevier, 2016

Denniston A. K. O., P. I. Murray. *Oxford Handbook of Ophthalmology.* Oxford University Press, 2018.

Johnson L. N., M. L. Diehl, C. W. Hamm, D. N. Sommerville, G. F. Petroski. Differentiating optic disc edema from optic nerve head drusen on optical coherence tomography. *Arch Ophthalmol.* 127(1): 2009; 45–59.

10 Flashing Lights and Floaters

Bhavana Sharma

KEY POINTS

1. Floaters usually represent age related changes (liquefaction) of the vitreous
2. Floaters occur in 70% of the population
3. Acute onset flashing lights and floaters should undergo a dilated fundus examination

DIAGRAM OF ALGORITHM

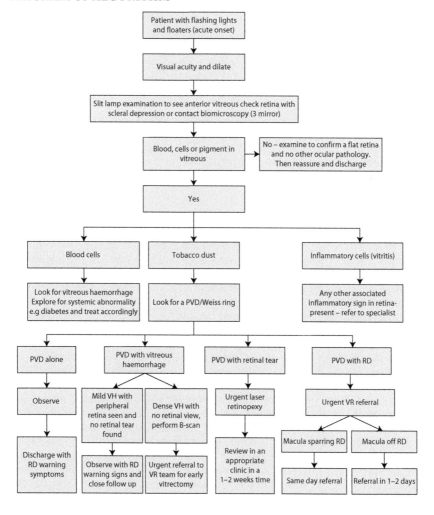

REFERRAL AND PRESENTATION

Flashing lights and floaters are one of the top presenting complaints a casualty officer will see. Patients tend to reach the urgent eye care service having first presented initially to their high street optometrist or very occasionally to A&E. If they have arrived having first been seen by their optometrist then they will have first dilated the patient and had a look and been worried for whatever reason and thus sent the patient in. It is unacceptable for optometrists to send patients in to the hospital with flashing lights and floaters without having dilated and properly examined the patient, and if they are unable to do this they should refer the patient to a competent optometrist who can. Accredited optometrists are usually very good at this and flashing lights and floaters are their bread and butter. If the patient has been to A&E first, the emergency doctor is almost certain to have performed a wholly inadequate examination as they lack the tools and skills to perform any meaningful examination. Patients almost never come from their general practitioners who nowadays don't see much of anybody with an eye problem and end up asking optometry to see them straight away.

See patients with symptoms of reduced vision or a fixed shadow urgently as they may have a retinal detachment. Alternatively, those with long standing floaters and normal vision can be reviewed by an optometrist.

Patients describe their symptoms with themes that have a common thread. They describe floaters as flies, cobwebs, worms, squiggly lines, strands or spots and so forth in their field of vision and find that these are more prominent against light coloured backgrounds like white walls or against a bright sky. These objects move with eye movement.

Flashing lights consist of sudden momentary arcs of light like a sudden flash of camera or bolt of lightning. Some people describe fireworks. They are more prominent in dim light and usually occur in the temporal field of vision and on eye movement. Both flashes and floaters do not involve loss of vision or the loss of field of vision. There is no pain.

DIFFERENTIAL DIAGNOSIS

Floaters and flashing lights don't have a long list of differential diagnoses. By far the commonest cause of floaters is syneresis. This is age-related liquefaction of the vitreous in which the formerly translucent type 2 collagen breaks down and becomes visible. These are entirely innocuous and affect 70% of the population, including the author(s). Secondly, floaters can result from true debris in the vitreous gel, most commonly structural debris resulting from a posterior vitreous detachment, blood or inflammatory debris.

A vitreous detachment occurs when the ageing vitreous body, which is 4 mL in volume and occupies almost the entirety of the posterior segment, collapses forward and pulls its posterior aspect free from the retina. This can either be a smooth collapse with no retinal tears or haemorrhages, or the blood vessels and retina can be damaged in the separation, resulting in pigment and blood released into the vitreous cavity, and even parts of the retina itself in the form of an operculated tear. Blood and inflammatory debris from diabetes, infection or inflammation of the posterior segment may also cause floaters (see Chapter 14). Diabetic retinopathy is a common cause of posterior segment haemorrhage.

The commonest cause of a flashing light is when the retina is stimulated as the vitreous pulls away during a posterior vitreous detachment (PVD), resulting in the illusion of light. Migraine can also cause flashing lights though the illusion is very distinctive here, with jagged edge flashes termed 'fortification spectra' that grow or diminish in the field of vision with a scotoma that may be associated with an advancing or retreating edge. Mostly, but not always, this flashing light is then followed by a typical migrainous headache after about 10–20 minutes of flashing light. Other less common causes of flashing lights include optic neuritis, occipital or ocular tumours, transient ischaemic attacks (TIA), head trauma and rubbing of eyes (termed phosphenes).

When both flashing lights and floaters occur together PVD is the main differential diagnosis, with an important emphasis on checking for retinal tears and retinal detachment. This makes new onset flashing lights and floaters a condition that must be seen by an eye specialist as a matter of priority, though it is rare that the hospital ophthalmologist will be the first to see.

CLINICAL EXAMINATION

All patient with flashing lights and floaters must have their visual acuity measured and fundus examined dilated.

Vitreous: The anterior vitreous should always be examined to assess for the presence or absence of tobacco dust, blood, pigment or inflammatory cells.

Retina: The retina itself should ALWAYS be examined with a dilated pupil. It is impossible to perform an adequate examination of a patient with flashing lights and floaters in the eye casualty without dilating them, no matter how close you are to running late. Ideally, a complete dilated examination must be carried out with indirect ophthalmoscopy and scleral indentation, though in practice this is such a palaver that usually contact lens biomicroscopy is undertaken using a 3-mirror lens or suitable widefield alternative, so as not to miss a peripheral break or tear.

A PVD itself can manifest as nothing more substantial than a few floaters accompanied by a mobile circular translucent floater somewhere overlying the optic disc, which is termed a Weiss ring (see Figure 10.1). If tobacco dust, motes of pigment in the anterior vitreous that move about on eye movement are revealed, the chance of a retinal tear or detachment being present has just risen substantially. This situation is discussed in detail in Chapter 16.

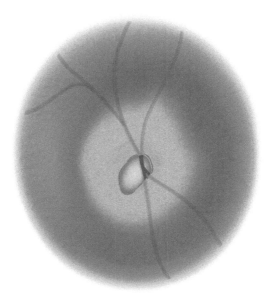

Figure 10.1 A posterior vitreous detachment with Weiss ring.

69

INVESTIGATIONS

If you are confident in the absence of any retinal tears or breaks, the absence of blood from any source of neovascularisation and inflammatory debris from vitritis and a PVD is evident, then this is a clinical diagnosis. If you are confident that your 3-mirror examination of the peripheral retina does not show anything remotely suggestive of a retinal tear or detachment then no further test or investigation need be performed. Usually the patient is given an information leaflet detailing warning signs, reassured and discharged.

B-scan: If however there is a compromised view of the fundus a B-scan ultrasound needs to be performed. This will not show any retinal tears unless they are either very large or the operator is particularly skilled, but even the lowliest ST1 will be able to spot a retinal detachment. This appears on B-scan ultrasonography as an extra line bulging into the cavity of the eye (see Figure 10.2).

RD vs Schisis: If a retinal detachment is thought to be potentially a retinoschisis, where the retina splits in two due to a degenerative process and is of infinitely less risk of progression, a few simple tests will help tell the difference. Firstly a retinoschisis produces an absolute scotoma overlying the affected area whereby a retinal detachment has only a relative scotoma. Retinoschisis tends to be bilateral and present temporally in hyperopes whereas retinal detachment is unilateral, can be present anywhere and is commoner in myopes. Retinoschisis is asymptomatic whereas a detachment has, well, flashing lights and floaters! Lastly a test with argon laser is useful whereby the ophthalmologist attempts to make a small laser burn over the suspicious area as you would with panretinal photocoagulation. It is possible in a retinoschisis and impossible in a detachment. OCT images over the raised area can also aid in the diagnosis, with schitic 'vertical bridging lines' being present in retinoschisis.

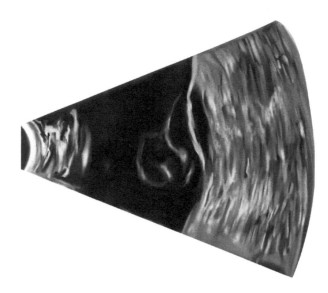

Figure 10.2 A B-scan ultrasound scan demonstrating a retinal detachment.

DIAGNOSIS

This is one of those areas of ophthalmology where raw clinical skill and appropriate use of bedside instruments can make all the difference here. The key is to have a high index of suspicion and to ALWAYS dilate patients presenting with these symptoms and to ALWAYS use a 3-mirror lens or suitable widefield alternative to check the peripheral retina. Let's face it, you're not going to try indirect ophthalmoscopy with indentation unless you have vitreoretinal aspirations. Use the history to direct your examination and the investigations above to diagnose syneresis, PVD, a retinal tear, a retinal detachment or any other cause for these symptoms. If you are unsure don't pass the buck by bringing the patient back to another session with another doctor; examine again and, if need be, ask a colleague or a senior to corroborate your findings.

MANAGEMENT

The key in dealing with patients presenting with flashing lights and floaters is to make the correct diagnosis. Once this is made the patient can be treated appropriately. Those patients with nothing at all to see can be reassured, and their symptoms blamed on syneresis if they have floaters or, depending on the nature of the flashing lights, migraine, be it ocular (with no headache) or classic (with a headache). If you are unsure but everything looks normal tell the patient this. Do not tell them they have a PVD if they do not have one; this creates great confusion should they then go on to have an actual PVD in future.

Posterior vitreous detachment: If the patient does have a PVD, then tell them to watch out for signs of a tear or detachment, usually a sudden new shower of floaters, new flashing lights, or a 'curtain/shadow' creeping across their vision. If your department has patient information leaflets with all this written down, ideally along with a contact number the patient should use should they experience any problem, then the patient can be discharged with advice.

Retinal tear: Any tobacco dust or blood, without sign of diabetic retinopathy or any other source of neovascularisation, needs to have a very extensive search performed for retinal tears or detachments. Should either of these be present refer to Chapter 16 for more information. Essentially immediate handover to the vitreoretinal team is needed in the case of a retinal detachment, with a macula on retinal detachment assuming the highest possible status of urgency. Retinal tears must be lasered as soon as possible and ideally by yourself should there be nobody else to do it there and then. The idea here is to prevent a retinal tear from developing into a retinal detachment. Have a low threshold to contact VR if you are unsure.

Retinal detachment: If there is a detachment present in the time it may take you to get the patient to the nearest VR unit, the patient can be asked to position their head in a particular way to prevent further progression of retinal detachment, especially in cases of macula on detachment. The patients are positioned on the side where the RD is mainly located. For example, a detachment located in the superior quadrant should be positioned supine, patients with detachment in the temporal quadrant should be positioned on the temporal side of the affected eye, patients with detachment in the nasal quadrant should be positioned on the nasal side and patients with inferior detachment are told to position upright.

Others: If the patient has signs of posterior inflammation responsible for the symptomatology turn to Chapter 14. If the patient is diabetic and the floaters are in fact caused by a haemorrhage, urgent panretinal photocoagulation (PRP) is the order of the day, and this needs to be arranged as a matter of priority, ideally to take place within a week and most certainly by 2 weeks. If there is any doubt in your mind that this will take place, it may be safer to perform the first lot of PRP immediately, but this should not be encouraged as the eye casualty is usually way, way too busy an environment to be able to do this comfortably. It is the duty of the medical retina consultants in that unit to ensure a system of robust handover of patients needing PRP from eye casualty to medical retina is in place.

FOLLOW UP

Discharge: Patients with syneresis or PVD do not need to be followed up. Give them a leaflet and discharge them. Consider review of high risk patients such as those with Sticklers and other high myopes.

Haemorrhagic PVD: The only exception whereby people with flashing lights and floaters are followed up in eye casualty is when a so called 'haemorrhagic PVD' is present and a few red blood cells are released at the time of the PVD, without causing an actual tear. These patients are sometimes seen for the sake of reassurance after a week, and re-examined, though if a confident examination is conducted initially this should not strictly speaking be necessary.

Tears: Patients with a retinal tear if not passed to the VR team for definitive management need to be referred after you have performed the laser yourself. Practice differs locally, with some VR surgeons preferring to follow up all lasered tears once, 2–3 weeks after the event, and others preferring primary discharge from eye casualty with follow up on an SOS basis. There is after all a 3%–4% rate of new tears again occurring in the weeks following first presentation with the initial retinal tear. Retinal detachment is immediately referred to VR and never followed up in eye casualty.

PITFALLS

1. The biggest pitfall is not dilating patients with flashing lights and floaters. Always do so. It is absolutely negligent not to.
2. Not using a 3-mirror, widefield or indirect ophthalmoscope to explore the periphery. That is a sure fire way to miss a tear or detachment.
3. Ignoring the presence of pigment in the vitreous – it is highly likely there is a tear.
4. Not safety netting your patients – document and give them retinal detachment warning signs.
5. Not explaining that floaters may remain – the patient may return assuming they would go!

FURTHER READING

American Academy of Ophthalmology Retina/Vitreous panel. *Preferred Practice Pattern Guidelines. Posterior Vitreous Detachment, Retina Breaks, and Lattice Degeneration.* San Francisco, CA: American Academy of Ophthalmology, 2014.

11 New Haemorrhages in the Vitreous and/or Retina

Tafadzwa Young-Zvandasara

KEY POINTS
1. Haemorrhages in the vitreous can present a diagnostic dilemma
2. B-scan ultrasound scan is a must in any obscured vitreous cavity
3. Retinal haemorrhages could be a sign of systemic disease
4. Be suspicious of an occult retinal tear in a vitreous haemorrhage especially when tobacco dust or a posterior vitreous detachment (PVD) is present

DIAGRAM OF ALGORITHM: VITREOUS HAEMORRHAGE

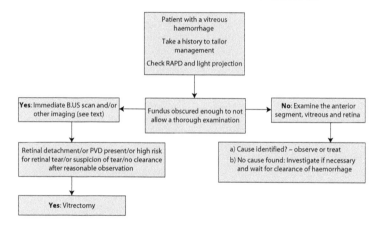

DIAGRAM OF ALGORITHM: RETINAL HAEMORRHAGE

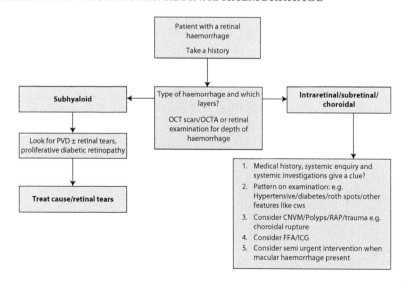

REFERRAL AND PRESENTATION

Typically these patients present with painless loss of vision in one eye, with the presence or absence of a shower of floaters that may well be red in colour.

Vitreous haemorrhage: A vitreous haemorrhage can present a diagnostic dilemma; it could be an innocuous feature which will resolve or may be part of a sight threatening and, very rarely, life threatening process. It is important to quickly decide which cases are harbouring a threat.

Retinal haemorrhage: Retinal haemorrhages may be due to systemic disease, and investigations may help establish an important underlying diagnosis.

DIFFERENTIAL DIAGNOSIS

Listing all the potential causes of a vitreous haemorrhage is an arduous task. It is more important to appreciate the unique relationship of the vitreous humour, vitreous cavity and the retina. Do take the individual presentation in context, and a thorough history and examination will direct your investigations and management.

Any source of haemorrhage may fill the vitreous cavity; including iris and ciliary body lesions. Examples of iris causes include trauma, iatrogenic causes, iris tufts and neovascularisation of the iris (see Figure 11.1), tumours, malignancy and idiopathic causes, etc. This list is similar for ciliary body causes and also includes iatrogenic causes such as poor pars plana entry during intravitreal injections. Retinal haemorrhages can result in a 'breakthrough' bleed into the vitreous cavity. Even more worrying is a retinal haemorrhage obscuring a decent retinal examination in a patient with a recent posterior vitreous detachment (PVD). The urgency is ruling out an underlying retinal tear or a retinal detachment.

Retinal detachments: Might be discernible on an ultrasound B-scan, *but one should never exclude a retinal tear based on US findings, and similarly diagnosing a tear on an US is difficult.* The blood in the vitreous cavity is a cause of proliferative vitreoretinopathy (PVR) based retinal detachment, which is classically tractional as opposed to rhegmatogenous, though could be mixed if the former leads to the latter. When suspicions of a tear arise, it is prudent to deal with these patients at the retinal tear stage by performing an urgent vitrectomy and exploration.

Vitreous haemorrhage: The list is long: PVD with or without a tear, retinal detachment; retinal pathology such as age related macular degeneration with CNVM,

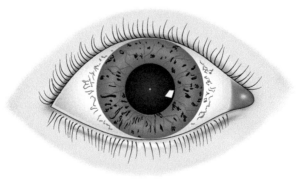

Figure 11.1   Iris neovascularisation in the presence of proliferative retinopathy.

idiopathic polypoidal choroidal vasculopathy, retinal angiomatous proliferation, macroaneurysms, CRVO/BRVO and diabetic retinopathy. Other causes of haemorrhage include neovascularisation which may be due to sickle, ROP, Eales, radiation, ocular ischaemic syndrome, Terson's syndrome, rarely, adult and juvenile X-linked retinoschisis, trauma (including laser injuries), iatrogenic causes and malignancy such as leukaemia. Always consider masquerades and other rare causes.

Retinal haemorrhage: Vitreous haemorrhage can originate from the retina as above (breakthrough haemorrhage). Also consider other causes such as hypertension, trauma (with or without choroidal rupture), head trauma, abusive head trauma, malignancy (leukaemia, lymphoma and so on), hypertension, infections (HIV, CMV, HZO/HSV, TB, toxoplasma, toxocara), any cause of traction on the retina, any cause of retinopathy such as sickle, valsava, radiation, Eales disease, hypoxia and barotrauma. Macular haemorrhage poses a risk to the macula. It may cause toxicity. Consider early intervention to displace haemorrhage away from the macular.

CLINICAL EXAMINATION

Take a careful history and perform all the necessary steps of an ophthalmic examination. Also check the pupillary responses, including RAPD for prognosis, light appreciation/projection in all four quadrants to detect the area of a potential retinal detachment (when unable to obtain a fundal view). Consider the context of presentation, in the case of trauma, ensure the globe is intact and absence of an intraocular foreign body (IOFB) if not.

It can be helpful to localise the level of the retinal haemorrhage for both diagnostic and management purposes. The level of haemorrhage may be evident on clinical examination by looking for the location of blood in relation to a blood vessel for example. This may be vitreal, subhyaloid, intraretinal, subretinal (between photoreceptors and RPE) or choroidal (see Figure 11.2). The haemorrhage may also be present in multiple layers.

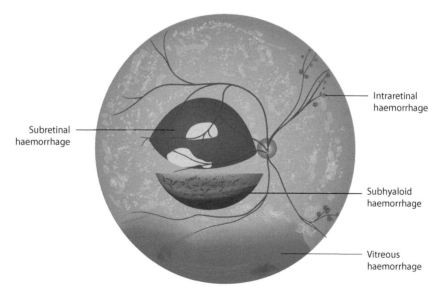

Figure 11.2 Examples of vitreal, subhyaloid, intraretinal and subretinal haemorrhages.

INVESTIGATIONS

Vitreous haemorrhage/retinal haemorrhage: A B-scan US is usually all that is required in addition to slit lamp examination to further image an eye with vitreous haemorrhage. Consider bloods including INR, OCT, FFA or ICG for diagnostic/prognostic/treatment purposes or if masquerades are suspected, but good reason would have to be present to order these from eye casualty. Do not forget routine clinic tests: BP, temperature, pulse and urinalysis where indicated.

A CT scan or MRI might be considered in trauma cases or when you are suspecting malignancy or other similar pathology. Avoid MRI when a metallic intraocular foreign body (IOFB) is suspected.

DIAGNOSIS

This is clinical. See text above for the causes of vitreous and retinal haemorrhages.

MANAGEMENT

Vitreous haemorrhage: If PRP for PDR, or retinopexy for a tear, cannot be adequately performed due to poor view then VR referral is required. See Chapter 16 for the management of retinal tears/detachment.

Urgent: In cases of vitreous haemorrhage, urgent vitrectomy is required if you suspect a retinal tear, PVD ± tear or retinal detachment. This is because time is precious, and a tear might lead to a retinal detachment and subsequent permanent damage to vision. When a single tear is visible with a vitreous haemorrhage and laser cannot be applied, cryotherapy might be sufficient. If not possible a vitrectomy can also be performed in this situation, though these are problems for the VR team to solve and not yourself; refer onwards and see the next patient.

Semi urgent: Vitrectomy for laser naïve type 1 diabetics, other non-immediate sight threatening pathology. Vitrectomy ± tPA and gas tamponade within 14 days for large submacular haemorrhages; this is suggested to prevent scarring.

Less urgent: Vitrectomy for persistent vitreous haemorrhage, treated diabetics – 6 to 8 weeks and consideration of anti-VEGF injections. This should not be a rule and should be dependent on the presentation or risk factors discussed already. CNV secondary to macular degeneration needs to be seen and treated within 2 weeks for example.

Observation: If the fundus and periphery are clearly visualised and sight/life threatening pathology ruled out then the patient can be observed for signs of improvement. It must be stressed, however, that eye casualty is not the place for this as a rule; it is not unheard of sadly for a patients with a non-resolving vitreous haemorrhage to be followed up there for weeks until eventually a macular off retinal detachment occurs.

Retinal haemorrhages or non-fundus obscuring vitreous haemorrhage: Treat the cause if identified, e.g. PRP, sectoral laser, direct laser to retinal macroaneurysms, PDT or anti VEGF injections. These interventions are not undertaken typically in eye casualty with the exception of possibly PRP, where a delay in clinic follow up may put a patient at risk of a worse haemorrhage than that already present.

FOLLOW UP

Vitreous haemorrhage: Serial B-scan ultrasound when the fundus is not adequately visualised and a tear/RD is not suspected. Frequency of follow up is determined by the suspicion about the cause of the haemorrhage and some advocate a minimum of weekly visits, though again this should not be in eye casualty. This should be continued until the retina is visualised clearly and pathology excluded. With the improved safety of vitreoretinal surgery, VR surgeons now intervene earlier, so speak to your local VR surgeon for advice. Diabetics need expedited review in a few weeks for resolution; those with no prior PRP need urgent referral.

Retinal haemorrhage: Find the cause and investigate. Referral to other specialties or multi-disciplinary team might be necessary.

PITFALLS

1. Not considering a retinal tear to be present in a case with a vitreous haemorrhage.
2. Not performing a B-scan ultrasound when the fundal view is diminished; this applies to even cases where some of the fundus is visualised.
3. Retinal haemorrhages due to systemic causes usually have a pattern which can give clues about the cause such as their location and extent. Do not forget to do simple clinic investigations such as BP and urinalysis to identify risk factors and check for an RAPD.
4. Always remember to tell the patient to return if symptoms become worse – the patient with the haemorrhage due to suspected PVD may develop (or you may have missed) a tear/RD elsewhere.
5. Not checking an INR in a patient on warfarin with a vitreous haemorrhage.

---

12 There is Something Strange and Unusual at the Back of the Eye

Rhianon Perrott-Reynolds

KEY POINTS

1. Patients may be entirely asymptomatic but very anxious
2. Involve the responsible consultant as soon as possible
3. An anterior segment examination and IOP check is essential
4. Remember to image extensively

DIAGRAM OF ALGORITHM

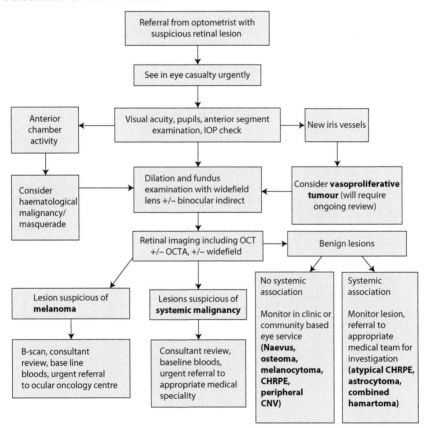

REFERRAL AND PRESENTATION

Unless there is a significant amount of exudation from the lesion in question, or proximity to the macula is an issue, there is very likely to be virtually no symptoms associated with the more unusual posterior pole findings. Often the patient pitches up at the emergency clinic after being referred from their optometrist when they had simply popped in to update their spectacles. This lack of symptoms firstly means that it is difficult to determine a duration and also means that the patient has been potentially thrust into a terrifying situation for them where the optometrist is not happy with what they've seen but at the same time cannot give them a diagnosis beyond 'I need someone to look at this very quickly'. Fortunately, the outcome is not often such that the services of the ocular oncology service need to be sought.

If symptoms are present, they are often vague and non-specific such as photopsia, photophobia, a non-descript discomfort in the eye or floaters if there is vitreous involvement.

There may be a drop in vision if there is sub retinal fluid or a lesion encroaching on the macula or if the suspicious lesion has bled causing a vitreous haemorrhage stopping the patient seeing out and you seeing in.

DIFFERENTIAL DIAGNOSIS

Obviously the first thing that jumps to mind when there is something strange and unusual at the back of the eye, is cancer. Whilst this is an obvious concern it is not always the case (see Table 12.1 for a list of choroidal and retinal tumours). Often a suspicious lesion turns out to be a simple naevus rather than the much more worrying melanoma.

A naevus is generally relatively well defined and flat, of varying sizes, often with a depigmented halo. Overlying drusen are a reassuring feature (see Figure 12.1). Naevi are present in 5%–10% of Caucasians and rarer in darker skinned individuals. The lifetime risk of malignant transformation is only around 1%, and these can happily be monitored on an annual basis in a community by optometrists with imaging facilities.

A choroidal melanoma on the other hand, tends to be less well defined and raised, often dome like in nature (see Figure 12.2). It may be pigmented but then again it may be amelanotic and appear pale or white. Often there may be associated subtle sub retinal fluid or an extensive exudative detachment. Overlying orange pigment called lipofuscin, incompletely digested photoreceptor outer segments – a mix of lipids, proteins, and fluorescent compounds is indicative of a melanoma.

Other choroidal lesions of a worrying nature include metastasis from a systemic malignancy. Solid lesions tend to be multiple and creamy white in nature, very

Table 12.1: **An Organisation of Posterior Pole Tumours**

Choroidal tumours

Malignant	Benign	Other
Melanoma	Naevus	Peripheral CNV
Choroidal metastisis	Osteoma	
Lymphoma	Melatonocytoma	
	Haemongioma	

Retinal lesions

Vascular	Hamartomas
Capillary haemangioma	Typical CHRPE
Cavernous haemangioma	Atypical CHRPE
	Combined hamartoma of the retina and RPE
	Astrocytoma

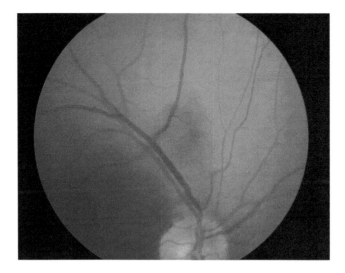

Figure 12.1 A typical choroidal naevus. (Courtesy of Miss Susmita Bala, Consultant Ophthalmologist, Queens Medical Center, Nottingham, UK.)

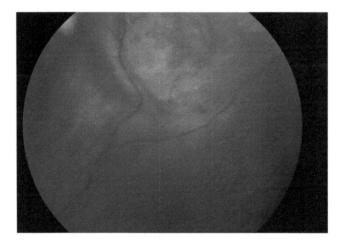

Figure 12.2 A choroidal melanoma. (Courtesy of Miss Susmita Bala, Consultant Ophthalmologist, Queens Medical Center, Nottingham, UK.)

much larger than seen in white dot syndromes and as such are difficult to confuse with one another. Unlike melanoma, metastases tend to be flatter, exude fluid, and may demonstrate RPE clumps. The most common primary sites are the breasts in women and the lungs in men.

Haematological malignancies also spread to the eye and tend to involve the whole eye in some way. Leukaemia often demonstrates a haemorrhagic infiltration with multiple lesions. Vitreous cells and hypopyon or more correctly a pseudo-hypopyon are seen. Lymphoma also has vitreous and anterior chamber involvement and can be mistaken for a chronic uveitis and hence falls in the 'masquerade' category. Posterior pole shows multiple creamy white lesions, generally smaller than that seen in metastasis – often termed leopard spots.

Occasionally you may be asked to see a young child with a white reflex suspicious of a retinoblastoma. These are fast growing white retinal lesions which may be unilateral, or if there is a family history, bilateral. Due to the complex emotional issues and examination difficulties in such cases these are best managed by the paediatric ophthalmologist who should be involved as soon as feasibly possible, and should ideally bypass the eye casualty setting all together (See Chapter 19).

Less worrying diagnosis of choroidal tumours include osteoma, haemagnioma and melanocytoma.

Choroidal osteomas are benign lesions that undergo ossification (calcium deposition). They tend to be well circumscribed creamy or placoid lesions, usually singular and often relatively close to the disc. Investigations including an ultrasound as these lesions are characteristically very hyperreflective.

Haemangiomas appear as indistinct orange oval masses with no lipofuscin and show a well-defined solid lesion with no shadowing on B-scan imaging. These lesions are generally inactive and cause no issues throughout life. Occasionally they may have some associated subretinal fluid which may cause a drop in vision if the macula is involved. Melanocytomas are densely pigmented lesions appearing almost completely black often seen at the optic disc, but can involve any aspect of the choroid. They are generally benign and do not require any intervention.

Occasionally a peripheral disciform or choroidal neovascular membrane may be sent in as a suspicious lesion. These extra foveal lesions occur very much less frequently than the more common macula CNV, but may appear almost identical. Fortunately, as long as the macula is not involved treatment is not indicated.

Other lesions which may cause suspicion are those originating from the retina. Fortunately these tend not to be malignant in their own right but may be a manifestation of a systemic condition. These include vascular tumours and hamartomas. There are four types of vascular tumours: capillary haemangioma, cavernous haemangioma, retinal arteriovenous communication and vasoproliferative tumours.

Capillary haemangiomas are associated with von Hippel-Lindau in 40% of cases. They begin as small red dots and grow into a vascular mass with feeder and draining vessels that might exhibit subretinal exudation or fibrosis. As long as the patients are symptom free no treatment is needed, although occasional treatment may be needed in troublesome situations.

Cavernous haemangiomas look more like a bunch of purple grapes with no obvious feeder/draining vessels and in general cause no problems and need no treatment. They can however be associated with skin haemangiomas and cerebral aneurysms, so it is not unreasonable to undertake neurological investigation or imaging to exclude this, but again this need not be ordered from eye casualty itself.

Arteriovenous malformation is also known as racemose haemangioma and is a benign lesion that does not generally require treatment. There may be a mass of abnormal vessels akin to a group of earthworms, and may in rare cases be associated with mid brain lesions in Wyburn–Mason syndrome.

Retinal vasoproliferative tumours tend to have a worse prognostic outcome in terms of vision and potential for complication than the other vascular tumours. They start as single or multiple creamy nodules in the peripheral retina. They can produce marked amounts of exudation that can extend to the macula and cause visual loss, which is difficult to reverse. They can be associated with retinal detachment and neovascular glaucoma, and can be difficult to differentiate clinically from other tumours including choroidal melanoma, so careful work up is needed.

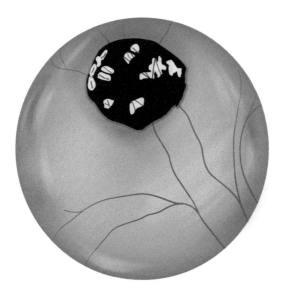

Figure 12.3   Congenital hamartoma of the retinal pigment epithelium.

Retinal hamartomas are begin lesions but can be associated with a systemic condition. The most common is congenital hypertrophy of the RPE or CHRPE. A lesion often referred as possible melanoma is the completely harmless 'typical' CHRPE, which is a purely incidental, inconsequential finding. These are well defined, pigmented round and flat. They may be solitary, multiple or present in a very pretty bear track pattern, however all are harmless (see Figure 12.3).

An 'atypical' CHRPE, however, may need investigation by a friendly gastroenterologist due to its association with Gardener's syndrome and colonic carcinoma. These atypical CHRPE lesions are normally greater than four in number and variable in shape and may have findings such as a comet or fish tail-like appearance.

A combined hamartoma of the retina and RPE can at first glance cause a concern of a nasty malignancy; however, in itself it is a harmless finding. It is often associated with neurofibromatosis and if found in a child without such a diagnosis, they should be referred to a paediatrician to investigate further. These lesions have a fibrous looking appearance with pigment and vascular tissue – a bit of everything. However they tend to be well defined and vision is maintained unless the fovea is involved.

Astrocytoma is a tumour associated with tuberous sclerosis (TS). It looks like a creamy white nodular mass, like a small rice pudding. It may cause vision loss by CNV or vitreous haemorrhage but does not require treatment unless these occur; however, they do need a systemic work up for other manifestations of TS.

CLINICAL EXAMINATION

As with all examinations of the eye, acuity is essential, visual fields may also be useful if loss of field is a complaint, and it is always a good idea to have a look at what the pupils are doing. Some unusual conditions may manifest with signs throughout the eye such as ocular lymphoma, which may persist with a low grade anterior uveitis that is not responsive to steroids and some vitreous changes such as sheets of cells. It is therefore essential to perform a good anterior segment examination before charging towards the posterior pole where you are expecting to see something. Neovascular glaucoma is also a possible complication of some of these conditions and so a good look for new iris vessels and an IOP are also suggested.

The posterior pole examination has to be done with a good level of dilation so both tropicamide and phenylephrine should be used. Do not be tempted to try to examine without dilation if the patient may have driven to the appointment and requested not to be dilated. You will need to explain to them that is an essential part of the examination and given the information provided by the optometrist, delay in a full examination should not be made. Fundus examination should be made with the widest field lens you have available, and you may want to use a three mirror if you are comfortable doing so. However many of the modern lenses give a field of view comparable to three mirror lens without the discomfort for the patient of a contact lens. One thing you should not be tempted to do is indent, as this may cause peripherally located tumours to bleed. If the lesion is large then using a binocular indirect headset is often an excellent way to determine the extent of the lesion.

INVESTIGATIONS

Within the casualty setting investigation will be mainly limited to imaging modalities. A standard retinal photograph or widefield imaging is essential for both effective onward referral if needed and monitoring purposes. Certainly an OCT of the lesion can be useful if you have a skilled photographer who can reach beyond the normal macula or optic nerve head scan, which may demonstrate subretinal fluid (SRF). OCT angiography can also be useful as it can show an abnormal vasculature without the invasive use of imaging contrast and can be done swiftly within the eye casualty setting.

Traditional dye based imaging of fluorescein angiography or ICG are of limited value in differentiating a naevus from a melanoma with no standard pathognomonic pattern. In some cases a dual circulation may be seen and ICG may give a more true representation of the extent of the lesion. Where these techniques may be useful are in the differentiation of similar looking lesions such as haemangioma or an extra foveal neovascular membrane. Fundus autofluorescence is a technique often forgotten; however, it can be very useful in showing up subtle lipofuscin which will be intensely hyperautofluorescent, which can aid in the diagnosis of melanoma.

A B-scan ultrasound will lend information that will often lead you towards making a diagnosis. Lesions which demonstrate a height of greater than 2 mm with a homogenous or solid appearance and a shadow behind, termed acoustic hollowing, are generally indicative of a choroidal melanoma. An osteoma will have a bright reflective appearance consistent with the high calcium content of the lesion.

Blood tests should be focused towards looking for a systemic disease and include standard full blood count, liver enzyme and renal function when a malignancy is suspected. There is little value in other tests at this point, and even if a metastatic cause is possible focused assessment is better done by an oncology specialist.

DIAGNOSIS

Diagnosis of these conditions may not be made immediately in eye casualty. Some are very obvious such as many naevi, haemagiomas and hamartomas and do not require any further intervention other than referral into the outpatient clinic for monitoring. Some can be discharged directly such as a typical CHRPE, with pictures. However many will not be clear cut and require further investigation and senior review and occasional highly specialised review to come to a final diagnosis.

MANAGEMENT

Again management is unlikely to be carried out in the casualty setting and will range from discharging the patient with an urgent referral to an ocular oncology unit or other medical specialties. The role of the emergency doctor here is simply to recognise the issue and refer onward. It is useful to be in a position to tell the patient roughly what to expect and that you would like a second opinion about the lesion that you deem suspicious.

FOLLOW UP

As with management, follow-up is dependent on the ultimate diagnosis; however, it is quite clear that these patients should not be followed up in eye casualty. In some places patients that are discharged can be given a copy of their photographs to be shared with their optometrist for comparison.

PITFALLS

The main pitfall is not identifying a dangerous, sinister pathology and not involving the consultant responsible for the patient at the earliest opportunity. Others are not carrying out a full examination and missing subtle signs such as anterior chamber cells or early iris new vessels.

FURTHER READING

Bowling B. *Kanski's Clinical Ophthalmology: A Systematic Approach*; 8th ed. Elsevier Health Sciences, 2015.

Sundaram V., A. Barsam, L. Barker, P. T. Khaw. *OST Training in Ophthalmology: The Essential Clinical Curriculum*; 2nd ed. OUP Oxford, 2016.

The Royal College of Ophthalmologists. Referral pathways for adult ocular tumours. https://www.rcophth.ac.uk/wp-content/uploads/2017/09/Referral-pathways-for-adult-ocular-tumours-June-2017.pdf

13 Wavy Lines, Distorted Vision and Blur

Annie See Wah Tung

KEY POINTS

1. Try to obtain a detailed description of symptoms. Patients may be vague and not produce textbook descriptions of symptoms.
2. Some macular changes can be subtle. Optical coherent topography is invaluable in detecting and diagnosing macular disorders.

DIAGRAM OF ALGORITHM

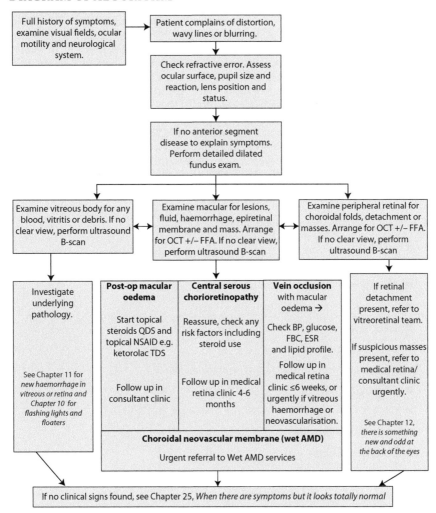

Full history of symptoms, examine visual fields, ocular motility and neurological system. → Patient complains of distortion, wavy lines or blurring.

Check refractive error. Assess ocular surface, pupil size and reaction, lens position and status.

If no anterior segment disease to explain symptoms. Perform detailed dilated fundus exam.

Examine vitreous body for any blood, vitritis or debris. If no clear view, perform ultrasound B-scan ↔ Examine macular for lesions, fluid, haemorrhage, epiretinal membrane and mass. Arrange for OCT +/− FFA. If no clear view, perform ultrasound B-scan ↔ Examine peripheral retinal for choroidal folds, detachment or masses. Arrange for OCT +/− FFA. If no clear view, perform ultrasound B-scan

Investigate underlying pathology.

See Chapter 11 for *new haemorrhage in vitreous or retina and Chapter 10 for flashing lights and floaters*

Post-op macular oedema	**Central serous chorioretinopathy**	**Vein occlusion** with macular oedema →
Start topical steroids QDS and topical NSAID e.g. ketorolac TDS	Reassure, check any risk factors including steroid use	Check BP, glucose, FBC, ESR and lipid profile.
Follow up in consultant clinic	Follow up in medical retina clinic 4-6 months	Follow up in medical retina clinic ≤6 weeks, or urgently if vitreous haemorrhage or neovascularisation.

Choroidal neovascular membrane (wet AMD)

Urgent referral to Wet AMD services

If retinal detachment present, refer to vitreoretinal team.

If suspicious masses present, refer to medical retina/ consultant clinic urgently.

See Chapter 12, *there is something new and odd at the back of the eyes*

If no clinical signs found, see Chapter 25, *When there are symptoms but it looks totally normal*

REFERRAL AND PRESENTATION

Distortion and blurred vision are very common causes of an ophthalmology referral, but not all are emergencies. Understand what your patient's symptoms are. If a patient describes classic central distortion, it helps focus the location of pathology to the macula. The diagnosis is straightforward when you know what to look for. However, patients may describe vague symptoms such as 'things are not as clear as before', or 'my glasses are dirty but I can't get it clean'. If the symptoms were insidious and mild, patients may present to their optometrist, hoping a change of glasses may help solve their problem.

Most countries in the UK have a community based eye care system which is run by optometrists. In Wales, most of these patients would be seen under the Welsh Eye Care Scheme (WECS). After checking the patient's refractive error, a diligent optometrist would dilate the patient's pupils to examine their fundus.

If the history and clinical signs are in keeping with a known pathology, they are then directly referred to the wet age-related macular degeneration (AMD) service or macular clinic accordingly. However, macular changes can sometimes be subtle, and without the help of an OCT in the community, it is difficult to confirm diagnosis and hence assess the urgency of such cases. In fact, even when an OCT is performed optometrists may still not know what the abnormality found is, resulting in patients being referred to the emergency clinic for further investigation and assessment.

A careful history can help differentiate between the causes of visual disturbances. Are the symptoms monocular or binocular? Are the changes only occurring in certain parts of the field of vision or globally? Do they see a kink or wavy line when a straight line is present (metamorphopsia)? Or do objects appear larger/zoomed in (macropsia) or smaller/zoomed out (micropsia)? What is the onset of symptoms? Are there associated headaches or floaters or previous retinal pathology? Many causes of blurred vision are covered elsewhere in this book. In this chapter, I will be focusing on macular diseases causing distortion and blurred vision.

DIFFERENTIAL DIAGNOSIS

Corneal or anterior segment causes (blurring):

- Dry eyes
- Uveitis
- Keratoconus, corneal ulcer or thinning
- Mydriasis
- Cataracts
- Subluxed lens or IOL

Other posterior segment disease (blurring or distortion):

- Choroidal folds
- Choroidal masses
- Retinal detachment
- Posterior uveitis

Macular disease (blurring or distortion):

- Choroidal neovascular membrane
- Central serous retinopathy

- Macular oedema (vein occlusions, diabetic, post-operative, uveitic)
- Epiretinal membrane
- Macular holes or pseudo-hole

Other causes:

- Ocular migraine (distortion)
- Visual field defect (blur)
- Diplopia/nystagmus (blur)
- Other neurological conditions (distortion/blur)

CLINICAL EXAMINATION

Pre-slit lamp examination: Visual acuity should always be measured and documented and should be clearly written whether or not glasses are used. An improvement of vision with pinhole suggests there is an element of refractive error. Macular disorders would not produce an improvement with pinhole unless patient is fixating eccentrically. Near vision should ideally be tested as well in the case of myopia, but this is not usually feasible in a busy emergency clinic.

Anterior segment assessment: Any anterior segment disease has the potential of causing blurry vision. They are usually associated with other symptoms like redness, pain or photophobia. Patients with severe dry eyes or eyes that water excessively can both cause blurry vision. Painless blurry vision or reduced vision always requires a dilated fundus examination. If your patient describes intermittent blurry vision, assess their anterior chamber depth and perform gonioscopy prior to dilating, to rule out intermittent angle closure. A subluxed natural lens or de-centred intraocular lens (IOL) implant can cause a shift in focus and blurry vision. If an IOL is significantly de-centred, or the patient's pupils dilated, the edge of the lens would diffract light and cause distortion or an arc of light is seen in the peripheral vision. Detailed examination is required to see if the lens is still stable.

Posterior segment: After excluding cataract or vitreous causes of blurred vision, you can then move onto assess the fundus.

Macular haemorrhages: Come in all sorts of sizes, from small dot haemorrhages, to large subretinal/preretinal bleeds. Clues to their aetiology may be helped by looking at the fellow eye. If CNV due to wet AMD/myopia/uveitis is not suspected consider cardiovascular history (macroaneyrsms), valsalva and other trauma.

If there is macular haemorrhage in one eye, look for associated drusen (well defined white-yellowish extracellular deposits – see Figure 13.1) or a pigmented epithelial detachment (PED). If the patient is young and there are no signs of drusen, look for any signs of choroidal breaks, uveitis or a myopic fundus (pale tessellated fundus, tilted discs, chorioretinal atrophy).

Epiretinal membranes: Are fibrocellular structures that develop on the surface of the retina that may cause wrinkling or elevation of the inner retina. They can be seen as a yellowish sheen over the macular area, easily visible on OCT. Patients may be asymptomatic or complain of metamorphsia or blurring. Causes may be primary or secondary (look for signs of CRVO/uveitis/trauma/previous laser).

VMT and macular holes: At an early stage may simply present as a yellow spot or ring. As it develops, it may be seen as a central crescent shape defect, or at its

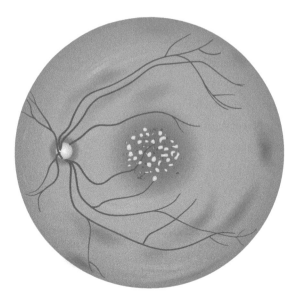

Figure 13.1 Macular drusen.

full-thickness form, a red base with yellow dots with surrounding cuff of greyish fluid – again, OCT is useful. Patient may be unaware of the deterioration of their sight as it is usually gradual.

Central serous retinopathy: In a young or middle-aged man (but not exclusively), with a well circumscribed raised macula area without haemorrhage, central serous retinopathy is likely. Patients typically describe blurring, metamorphopsia, micropsia or a central relative scotoma, have an A-type personality, are stressed or have a history of steroid use.

Macular oedema: Causes retinal thickening and loss of foveal reflex. You may also see cystoid appearance in the macula if there is significant cystic macular oedema (see Figure 13.2). If the patient is diabetic, changes are more likely to be bilateral

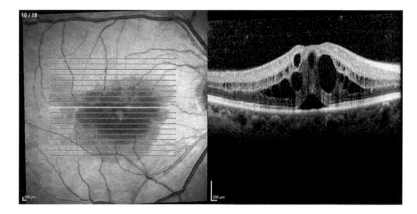

Figure 13.2 Cystoid macular oedema. (Courtesy of Miss Susmita Bala, Consultant Ophthalmologist, Queens Medical Center, Nottingham, UK.)

and may be associated with microaneurysms and exudations. In vein occlusions, there is accompanying dilatation and tortuosity of the venous circulation with a mixture of flame-shaped dot/blot haemorrhages. Cotton wool spots may also be present, or the patient may have undergone recent cataract surgery.

INVESTIGATIONS

Investigations can be divided into those that confirm diagnosis and those that identify risk factors. Consider requesting OCT imaging before you see the patient, so you are armed with suitable imaging to make an informed diagnosis in a timely manner.

Ocular imaging: An OCT image is most helpful in picking up any intra or sub-retinal fluid which will help confirm if there is a macular disorder. Macular oedema on OCT scanning shows retinal thickening with cystic hyporeflective spaces. AMD changes usually involve drusen deposition between retinal pigment epithelium and Bruch's membrane as well as a disruption of the retinal pigment epithelium. If there are blood vessels extending through Bruch's membrane then that is considered as choroidal neovascularisation (CNV). If CNV is associated with AMD changes, they do not usually require further investigation and would be treated under the wet AMD pathway. If the CNV is not associated with macular degeneration, other investigations may be required. Fundus fluorescein angiography and autofluorescence are useful in further confirming aetiology and areas of ischaemia in vein occlusions and diabetics, but are not required in the eye casualty setting.

Generally speaking, macular oedema is either due to inflammation, microvascular disease, vein occlusion or ischaemia. Other than taking a full medical history, you would want to check the patient's blood pressure, serum glucose, full blood count and erythrocyte sedimentation ratio (ESR). In a patient with vein occlusion who is less than 50 years of age, you may want to consider performing a clotting and vasculitis screening. However, this does not usually alter the treatment of macular oedema itself.

DIAGNOSIS

Diagnosis can be made clinically based on examination findings with OCT to help confirm the diagnosis. The most common conditions that cause distortion include choroidal neovascular membrane (CNV), epiretinal membrane and macular hole. There are various causes of CNV (see Table 13.1), and the patient's age and demographics can give you some clues.

Table 13.1: **Causes of Choroidal Neovascular Membrane**

Degenerative	Inflammatory
• Age related macular degeneration • Pathological myopia • Angioid streaks	• Presumed ocular histoplasmosis syndrome • Multifocal choroditis • Serpiginous choroidopathy • Bird-shot retinochoroidopathy • Punctate inner choroidopathy • Vogt–Koyanagi–Harada disease • Sarcodosis
Infectious	**Trauma**
• Toxoplasmosis • Tuberculosis • Lyme disease	• Choroidal rupture • Laser
Retinal dystrophies	**Idiopathic**
• Chorioretinal scars • Tumour	

Table 13.2: **Causes of Macular Oedema**

Inflammatory	Retinal vascular disease
• Posterior uveitis • Intermediate uveitis • Scleritis	• Diabetic macular oedema • Retinal vein occlusion • Ocular ischaemia • Retinal telangiectasia
Systemic	**Drug-induced**
• Hypertensive retinopathy • Chronic renal failure	• Topical progstagladin analogues e.g. latanoprost
Retinal dystrophies	**Degenerative**
• Retinitis pigmentosa	• Choroidal neovascularisation
Vitreous macular traction	**Tumour**
• Epiretinal membrane	• Retinal capillary haemangioma

Iatrogenic
  • Radiation retinopathy
  • Post-operative (cataract, corneal, vitreoretinal)
  • Post-cryotheraphy
  • Post-laser (peripheral iridotomy, panretinal photocoagulation)

Table 13.2 highlights causes of macular oedema. The patient's history and your ocular findings will help differentiate the cause although further investigations may help with atypical cases.

MANAGEMENT

Management in the acute setting would require treatment of abnormal risk factors such as high blood pressure for example. We as ophthalmologists rarely initiate systemic treatments for these cases, and it is best to ask the patient to attend their GP for ambulatory monitoring and commencement of treatment or the hospital medical team if significantly abnormal.

Macular oedema: The treatment of macular oedema occurs after onward referral to your medical retina service in the form of laser or injections. The decision of whether to treat with focal or grid laser, intravitreal anti-VEGF or peri-ocular steroid depends on the aetiology, amount of retinal fluid, patient factors and local policy. CMO after cataract surgery (Irvine–Gass syndrome) is initially treated with topical NSAIDs and steroids until review, though it is increasingly believed that the drops buy time at best for the eye to heal itself in most cases. Treatment for Irvine–Gass involves topical steroid with a topical non-steroidal drop (e.g. g. dexamethasone 1% QDS and g. ketorolac TDS). These patients should then be followed up in the consultant clinic.

CSR: Patients with central serous chorioretinopathy should be reassured that the majority of cases resolve spontaneously in 3–6 months. Risk factors including exogenous steroids used should be avoided if possible and avoidance of stress factors (where possible). If there is evidence of scarring from previous episodes or no resolution after 6 months, photodynamic therapy is sometimes used.

Wet AMD: Should be referred urgently through the relevant MR pathway within 2 weeks, with dry AMD discharged with advice. Most units now offer one-stop clinics where patients have an FFA, doctor's review and treatment involving an anti-VEGF intravitreal injection all within the same hospital visit.

Macular holes and epiretinal membranes: Should be referred to your vitreo-retinal service for consideration of surgery, if the patient would consider it. A full thickness macular hole generally requires surgery and should be referred to be seen within about 6 weeks or so, as the prognosis is affected by the duration of the morbidity, pre-operative vision and size of macular hole. Depending on patient's level of visual disturbance, visual acuity and rate of progression, epiretinal membranes do not always require treatment. The decision of treatment can be made by the patient with their vitreo-retinal surgeon after the discussion of the associated risk and benefits. Ideally these patients would be sent directly to VR services, avoiding the eye casualty if diagnosed by an optometrist in the community.

FOLLOW UP

All of the conditions discussed above should not require follow up in the emergency eye clinic. Many will require on-going treatment or monitoring with the medical/surgical retina teams.

PITFALLS

1. Co-pathology often exists. Choroidal neovascularisation can occasionally be associated with extensive lipid deposition which mimics diabetic macular oedema. On the other hand, a diabetic patient may present with subtle signs of a CNV resembling diabetic macular oedema. If there is sudden deterioration of vision, or if the visual acuity is not in keeping with the clinical course, perform an OCT scan to help your diagnosis, but check for an RAPD before dilating. Just because an epiretinal membrane is overlying an area of retinal thickening, it does not necessarily mean it is the cause of the oedema or reduced vision.
2. Optical coherence tomography must be interpreted with caution as well.
3. Remember to examine the peripheral retina, so as not to miss a growing melanoma.

FURTHER READING

Bowling B. *Kanski's Clinical Ophthalmology, A Systemic Approach*, 8th ed. 2016.

Dennison A., P. Murray. *Oxford Handbook of Ophthalmology*. Oxford University Press, 2014.

NICE Guideline. Age-related macular degeneration, 2018, https://www.nice.org.uk

Royal College of Ophthalmologists, Clinical Guidelines, Diabetic retinopathy, 2013. https://www.rcophth.ac.uk/wp-content/uploads/2014/12/2013-SCI-301-FINAL-DR-GUIDELINES-DEC-2012-updated-July-2013.pdf

Royal College of Ophthalmologists, Clinical Guidelines, Retinal vein occlusion (RVO), 2015. https://www.rcophth.ac.uk/wp-content/uploads/2015/07/Retinal-Vein-Occlusion-RVO-Guidelines-July-2015.pdf

14 Vitritis and Posterior Uveitis

Safa Ahmed Elhassan

KEY POINTS

1. Always dilate patients with anterior uveitis to examine the fundus
2. Any post-operative eye surgery patient should be considered to have infectious endophthalmitis in the immediate post-operative period
3. Time is short when it comes to treating acute retinal necrosis and infectious endophthalmitis
4. Involve senior clinicians as soon as possible in the management of sight threatening uveitis

DIAGRAM OF ALGORITHM

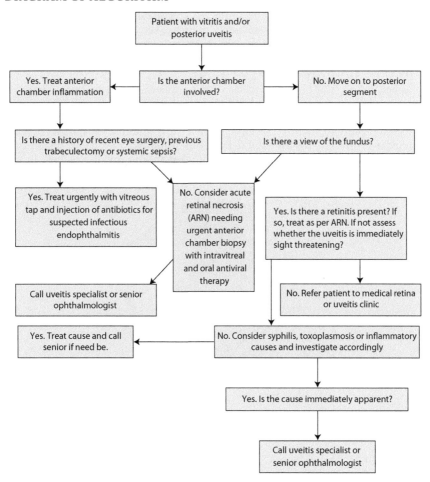

REFERRAL AND PRESENTATION

There are two main groups of patients that end up in this category: patients with a panuveitis and patients with a predominantly intermediate or posterior uveitis. This main distinction is important as the presentation is very different. Chapter 7 details how patients with anterior uveitis present, and the same mechanism brings in the same group of patients with panuveitis. Patients develop photophobia, a red eye and blurred vision, and it is this that brings them to the attention of ophthalmic services, either via the optometrist or via accident and emergency. As mentioned in that chapter multiple times, EVERY patient with anterior uveitis will need to be dilated to rule out a panuveitis. It is impossible to rule out any posterior element of inflammation without looking. Figure 14.1 outlines the three areas of the eye that get inflamed in anterior, intermediate and posterior uveitis. A panuveitis implies that every section of the uveal tract is inflamed.

Patients with panuveitis, detected after a patient with anterior uveitis is dilated, usually behave much the same in clinic as those with anterior uveitis alone. Patients with intermediate and posterior uveitis on the other hand present very differently. There is usually little to no photophobia or ciliary injection, and the main problem is actually blurred vision in the affected eye, sometimes with floaters. It is not unheard of for these patients to be picked up during routine optometry appointments and referred in because of unexpected findings at the back of the eye. These patients typically are a bit bewildered and are not entirely sure why they have suddenly been asked to come to see you, though there are those with very severe inflammation that are much more worried.

DIFFERENTIAL DIAGNOSIS

It is helpful to take both categories of patients one at a time here. There are certain conditions common to both that must be taken seriously for the risk of blindness is great. The first and foremost is acute retinal necrosis (ARN). This is a rapidly spreading viral infection of the retina that must be recognised immediately for any useful sight to be saved. Initially it may cause floaters and blur but this soon spreads to cause a significant anterior uveitis as well. In fact,

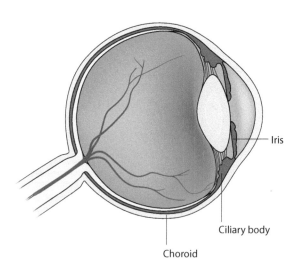

Iris

Ciliary body

Choroid

Figure 14.1 The different parts of the uveal tract most active in anterior, intermediate or posterior uveitis.

it is not uncommon for cases of ARN to first be misdiagnosed as an anterior uveitis alone. Secondly, endophthalmitis classically causes rip roaring anterior segment symptoms, but there is also equal if not more activity taking place behind the lens. Lastly in this group there are those patients with toxoplasmosis. Once these concerns have been addressed we can start considering the two groups of patients separately.

In the first group are the ones with good going anterior uveitis that have typical symptoms of this, as well as some posterior features such as vitritis, cystoid macular oedema (CMO) and perhaps retinal lesions. The differential diagnosis here, as well as those diagnoses in the common stem, includes a whole host of inflammatory diseases such as sarcoidosis, multifocal choroiditis, and infectious agents such as cat scratch disease and ocular tuberculosis. The list is immaterial to the casualty officer, and the only question you need to ask is: what do I need to do NOW.

The second group of patients have rip roaring anterior uveitis as well so you will definitely be doing something for that at least. The differentials here are stacked away from inflammatory conditions such as sarcoidosis, serpiginous and other less aggressive lesions and towards potentially devastating causes such as infections. Your role here is to recognise the difference and pass the patient on appropriately.

CLINICAL EXAMINATION

Visual acuity should be documented accurately and the patient then examined at the slit lamp. A history should be taken with specific emphasis on any recent eye surgery, a septic focus elsewhere, previous toxoplasmosis or immunosuppression from any cause. This should already be giving you clues before the patient's chin is yet rested on your chin rest.

The anterior chamber: Itself is either active or quiet, but take the time to measure cells and flare as documented in Chapter 7. Look also for keratic precipitates, posterior synechiae and measure the size of any hypopyon, if present.

IOP: It is essential to measure intraocular pressure (IOP) as uveitis of any cause can result in a pressure increase. Toxoplasmosis in particular causes a disproportionate rise in pressure and the IOP here can also be a clue as to the diagnosis.

Dilate: Once the state of the anterior chamber has been measured, dilate the patient. This really cannot be emphasised enough. Dilate every case of uveitis, regardless of the severity. It is negligent not to do so. Not only dilate the patient but also wait for the drops to work properly. Once this has been achieved first look at the anterior vitreous. Tilt the slit lamp and look under high magnification at the anterior vitreous, focusing just behind the lens, looking for debris and cells floating about.

Fundus: Next look at the posterior pole and macula. Are they visible? If there is absolutely no view whatsoever have a high index of suspicion for ARN, endophthalmitis, toxoplasmosis or syphilis. If they are visible, then look for a retinitis or signs of previous damage.

An acute retinitis looks like an area of whitened retina with a fluffy border (see Figure 14.2). Look for any other lesions that might suggest previous inflammation, with areas of scarring typically appearing as areas of pigment which may be punched out or raised. Toxoplasmosis typically appears as an area of reactivated retinitis at the border of an area of scarring. The macula should then be examined for potential cystoid macular oedema (CMO).

Lastly examine the peripheral retina for snowballs or snow banks that may indicate a predominantly intermediate uveitis, or for areas of peripheral scarring.

97

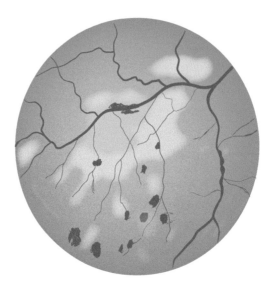

Figure 14.2 Acute retinal necrosis.

INVESTIGATIONS

As with anterior uveitis, less is definitely more when it comes to ordering investigations in the casualty room. Do what needs to be done and no more.

AC, vitreous tap: The first thing to ascertain is whether a sight threatening process is at play. If there is any suspicion of infectious endophthalmitis from recent eye surgery, or more rarely, a septic source elsewhere in the body, there is no time to delay whatsoever and an intravitreal tap for sampling with injection of antibiotics must be organised immediately. This must be done in a clean room or theatre, and the organisation of this will be fundamentally different in every hospital in the land so get acquainted with these procedures BEFORE the event so you know exactly what to do when the time comes. If the patient is septic then a blood culture can be taken in eye casualty straight away. If ARN is suspected then an anterior chamber tap for viral PCR sampling should be immediately undertaken and the form ticked so that HSV, VZV and CMV are all looked for.

Vitreous biopsy: Vitreous biopsy in some places is performed by the vitreoretinal team but much more commonly is undertaken by junior on call staff.

- The patient is prepared in a clean room or theatre and the eye anaesthetised with oxybuprocaine drops.

- 5% iodine is then applied to the conjunctival sac and the area prepared with 10% iodine to the skin prior to applying a sterile drape and speculum, as per cataract surgery.

- A 1 mL syringe attached to an orange needle is advanced into the vitreous 4 mm behind the limbus, perpendicular to the eye, and approximately 0.3 mL of fluid extracted.

  - Sometimes this is difficult and some movement (but not a lot!) is needed such as turning the bevel or angling the needle posteriorly but despite this, if no fluid is forthcoming change to a blue needle to get the sample.

- Occasionally this too will fail and the vitreoretinal team will need to be contacted.

■ Should a decent sample be obtained gently unscrew the needle from the syringe and use the same needle to inject your pre-prepared antibiotics.

- These should consist of vancomycin 1 mg in 0.1 mL and ceftazidime 2 mg in 0.1 mL. Get these prepared prior to the patient arriving in theatre as it usually takes a good 10–15 minutes to mix them up properly.

AC tap: An anterior chamber, or aqueous biopsy, can be undertaken at your slit lamp.

■ After preparation with topical anaesthetic and 5% iodine

■ Place a speculum and sit the patient at your slit lamp.

■ Using a grey needle attached to a 1 mL syringe advance into the anterior chamber just in front of the limbus, bevel toward you, and gently withdraw 0.1 mL of fluid. It is dangerous to take more.

Toxoplasmosis: Should toxoplasmosis be suspected then the diagnosis is usually clinical as the examination shows a 'headlight in the fog' appearance on fundoscopy as the active white lesion is visible behind the vitritis. Sometimes blood tests are undertaken for this in the form of toxoplasmosis IgM and IgG, but this is not really that useful in the eye casualty setting.

If a panuveitis of unknown cause is present and the fundus cannot be examined for clues, then plasma syphilis serology should be undertaken as well as viral PCR as per ARN.

If the patient has a vitritis picked up purely by chance and an intermediate uveitis is suspected, without significant anterior chamber inflammation, then it is best if the patient is plugged into the uveitis service.

Eye casualty officers are not experienced at uveitis and a common mistake is their ordering a billion blood tests and confusing the whole picture. If there is mild inflammation and no sight threatening pathology it is entirely reasonable to ask the uveitis service to pick the patient up and investigate accordingly.

DIAGNOSIS

If enough of the retina can be seen, ARN and toxoplasmosis can be diagnosed clinically, though confirmatory testing is essential in the former via an anterior chamber tap and PCR, with a posterior chamber sample taken if intravitreal Foscarnet is being considered.

Eye casualty is very busy, however, and sorting all this out takes a while so if possible it is best to decant this responsibility to someone else, be they an on call colleague or another ophthalmologist in training. If there is no other way then it must be done nonetheless, though it does mean a very long wait for those other patients waiting to see you. Do not be tempted to bring them back the next day; it might be too late to save any meaningful sight by then. If history and examination point toward infective endophthalmitis, then a vitreous sample with injection of antibiotics is a must and this cannot be escaped.

MANAGEMENT

Anterior uveitis in this situation is treated in exactly the same manner here as detailed in Chapter 7.

■ Infectious endophthalmitis needs immediate vitreous biopsy and injection of antibiotics.

- ARN is treated with aqueous biopsy and intravitreal Foscarnet 2.4 mg in 0.2 mL if available, with immediate commencement of oral Valaciclovir 2 g tds.

- If there is dense vitritis without an obvious cause then until the results of your aqueous and vitreous samples and serum syphilis test are back, it is reasonable to treat the patient with valaciclovir, azithromycin 500 mg od po (for toxoplasmosis) and potentially oral prednisolone 40–60 mg in the very short term to cover all bases.

  - In these cases, however, it is mandatory to speak to a senior and pass the patient on to a medical retina or uveitis specialist as SOON AS POSSIBLE.

If there is no anterior element of inflammation and the posterior element is old and picked up incidentally there is no rush; refer to your uveitis colleagues via formal outpatient referral. Less is more in this scenario.

FOLLOW UP

The work up of acute cases of catastrophic posterior inflammation is so time consuming and energy sapping that a single case can torpedo an entire casualty clinic. Investigation and immediate treatment is therefore best carried out by a medical retina or uveitis specialist immediately where possible. Follow up should therefore be arranged elsewhere from the outset. Should there be no such specialist immediately to hand, have a low threshold to admit the patient or at the very least arrange for them to be seen daily if there is no other way of decanting them to the correct team. Eye casualty isn't really the environment for these complicated patients, merely the entry point into the hospital system. Patients with incidental posterior uveitis should be followed by the uveitis team at the next arranged clinic and this arranged as per the usual mechanism at your institution. Again, follow up in eye casualty is not really ideal for these patients.

PITFALLS

1. Again, and always, the biggest pitfall is not dilating a patient with anterior uveitis for a look at the fundus. ALWAYS DILATE PATIENTS WITH ANTERIOR UVEITIS.
2. Missing ARN is another gigantic pitfall. This condition is rapidly blinding and without prompt action permanent visual damage can result. Time is short. Have a low threshold to suspect this, especially in immunocompromised patients.
3. Similarly missing infectious endophthalmitis is a terrible mistake. ANY post-operative eye surgery patient presenting with acute severe uveitis should be considered to have an infective cause, as should any patient that has had a trabeculectomy ever and any patient with septicaemia. Day 7–10 is the commonest time for post-operative endophthalmitis to first present.

FURTHER READING

Williams G. S., Westcott M. *Practical Uveitis: Understanding the Grape.* Taylor & Francis Group, 2017.

15 The Painful Eyeball

Alexander Kin Chiang Chiu

KEY POINTS

1. Pain is an associated symptom; history and examination is key
2. Always check pupil response and visual acuity to give you useful clues to the diagnosis
3. Pain of any level or severity may be the cause of patient attendance
4. Consider whether you need to check corneal sensation before instilling topical anaesthesia
5. Refrain from prescribing topical anaesthetics as a treatment from the eye casualty
6. Don't rely on the referring party's examination, always ask the right questions to rule out serious pathology

DIAGRAM OF ALGORITHM

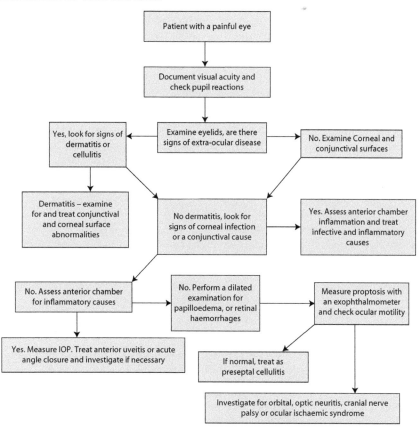

REFERRAL AND PRESENTATION

Pain is a common eye complaint and presents in different ways, causes of which can be differentiated by their accompanying symptoms. Pain may be experienced on the eye, behind the eye, in the eye and made worse with eye movement, on exposure to light, or on touch. Pain can be dull, sharp, or just be an annoying discomfort to the patient. Pain can be constant or intermittent. Varying degrees of pain can be problematic to one patient whereas another soldiers on. Pain can be proportionate with clinical signs and at other times you wonder what all the swearing is about. Vision may be affected with some due to media defects and others due to intense epiphora. Children in pain will be difficult to examine, their parents are usually distressed and your blood pressure will rise. Sensible use of topical anaesthetic will work wonders for your patient and yourself before you carry on examining the patient, and provision of a darkened room for them to wait in is a kindness.

You must always remember to be vigilant when seeing the patient because referrers can be wrong. General practitioners and A&E staff have little training in ophthalmology, coupled with limited ophthalmic resources; this results in them giving you a brief history with limited examination findings (usually with the VA upside down). Depending on the information gathered, a decision may be made of when to see the patient as you triage. It may even be prudent to ask them to send the patient to an accredited optometrist if they are unable to carry out a proper assessment for potentially a low risk pathology. The most helpful referrals tend to come from community optometrists such as those affiliated in Wales with the Welsh Eye Care Scheme (WECS) who are trained to perform a thorough ocular examination and refer urgent cases to you after they have themselves triaged and reviewed the patient armed with enough accurate information.

DIFFERENTIAL DIAGNOSIS

Differentials can be ordered based on the location of the pain or associated symptoms: photophobia or foreign body sensation with a red eye is commonly associated with anterior segment pathology, dull ache with visual disturbance – posterior scleritis, pain on eye movements with loss of vision – retrobulbar, diplopia and pain looking in one direction gaze – myositis or cellulitis, temporal tenderness – GCA.

Pain can be referred to the eye from adnexal, intracranial or facial structures such as the sinuses or teeth. If no obvious causes can be found, it is important not to forget asthenopic causes; uncorrected refractive error, phorias or tropias, convergence insufficiency, accommodative spasm and pharmacological causes. An orthoptist can help you with these.

The quality and severity of the pain can help locate and differentiate conditions: sharp stabbing nerve pains on the face and around the eye may precede a shingles rash, a dull ache keeping one up from sleep with a localised or general area of redness – scleritis versus episcleritis, mild discomfort with itching and grittiness may indicate allergy, dryness or blepharitis. Pain can be generalised or localised over the most tender point such as with dacryocycstitis, chalazia or scleritis.

See Table 15.1.

CLINICAL EXAMINATION

History: A clear history is essential to assess a painful eye including its duration, location, quality, severity and associated symptoms.

Examination: Visual acuity should always be performed prior to slit lamp examination. Pupil response is vitally important; a non-reactive pupil may indicate acute angle closure or iris Bombé; a blown out pupil may indicate trauma or cranial nerve palsy; a relative afferent pupillary defect may indicate optic neuritis. These

Table 15.1: Location of Pain and Common Associated Symptoms and Pathology

Location	Associated Symptoms	Differentials
Adnexal and face	Ache, localised pain	Periorbital causes of pain may be due to skin, sinus or dental related causes; preseptal cellulitis, dermatitis, dacryocystitis, referred pain, hordeolum or trauma. Orbital causes are less obvious to the eye, with these including idiopathic orbital inflammatory syndrome, orbital tumour or mass, optic neuritis, acute dacryoadenitis, migraine or cluster headache, diabetic cranial nerve palsy, sinusitis, trauma and orbital cellulitis.
Anterior segment	Foreign body sensation, epiphora, red eye, blurred vision, photophobia	Keratitis (from dry eye, infective causes, inflammatory, allergic, toxicity), keratoconjuntivitis (either infective or inflammatory), scleritis, corneal abrasions/lacerations, inflamed phlycten/pinguecula, or pterygium, foreign bodies, contact lens problems, post-operative infection/inflammation, anterior uveitis, endophthalmitis and acute angle closure glaucoma. Discomfort may be due to episcleritis, conjunctivitis or blepharitis
Orbit, muscles and nerve	Pain on eye movement, restricted eye movement and diplopia	Myositis, cellulitis, orbital fracture, retobulbar optic neuritis, orbital infiltration, tumour or haemorrhage.

are important signs that should not be missed and will aid the choice of adjunctive tests you need to perform.

Eyelids and eye movements: Examine the eyelids to rule out any obvious peri-orbital causes including dermatitis, pre-septal cellulitis, hordeolum or trauma. Mark around cellulitic areas to assess disease progression. Assess eye movements, orbital cellulitis, fracture and myositis would cause pain on eye movements with ocular motility examination displaying some signs of mechanical restriction with varying degrees of injection and oedema over the muscle.

External eye: The integrity of the conjunctival and corneal surfaces can then be assessed. Look for infiltrates, dendritic ulcers, foreign bodies, pinguecula, phlyecten or pterygia. Fluorescein dye can highlight severe meibomian gland disease or severe dry eye and demonstrate infiltrates and dendritic ulcers clearly. Corneal sensation is useful in differentiating between herpetic diseases and abrasions; remember to check this before instillation of topical anaesthetic.

Anterior chamber: Carefully look for signs of inflammation, blood, cells, flare or keratic precipitates. Hypopyon or hyphaema indicate a more severe infection, inflammation or trauma. This should be measured and documented for disease progression. Tonometry, either with a Goldmann tonometer or I-CARE is essential to manage the pressure in these cases and in general should be performed on all patients excluding cases of corneal perforation.

Posterior segment: Fundal examination should be attempted to identify a cause of the patient's pain if not identified already. Look for choroidal folds or effusions or optic disc abnormalities such as swelling, pallor or haemorrhages which may be associated with an orbital mass or infection, acute angle closure glaucoma or optic neuritis.

Associated ocular examination: Cover and uncover tests may be useful in determining the severity of phoria or tropias. Assess extraocular movements for identifying cranial nerve palsies or restriction. Use an exophthalmometer to measure proptosis.

INVESTIGATIONS

Not all investigations are necessary in all cases; they depend upon the history, clinical presentation and subsequently the differential diagnosis.

Swabs and scrapes: Corneal infections, abrasions and ocular surface disease are common causes of eye pain. Corneal scrapes and swabs may be indicated in severe infections involving large or odd corneal infiltrates, with infiltrates >1 mm potentially associated with anterior chamber involvement. Remember to swab recurrent or persistent cases of conjunctivitis (usually with follicles) for Chlamydia and keep a high suspicion for acanthamoeba in contact lens wears with poor hygiene.

Ocular imaging: Perform a B-scan ultrasound looking for possible posterior scleritis (T sign – see Figure 15.1). Optical coherence tomography is standard practice nowadays and is useful to image and assess the optic nerve and retina for painful pathology or associations.

Visual fields: Formal visual fields will be useful for optic neuritis cases or orbital tumours.

Systemic investigations: Cardiovascular risk factors including blood pressure (BP) need to be measured for cranial nerve palsies and ocular ischaemic syndromes. BP is important in cases of suspected papilloedema. If optic neuritis is suspected

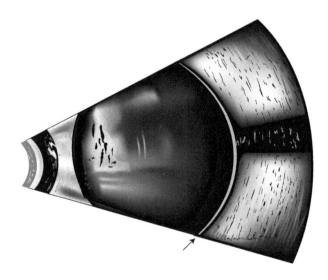

Figure 15.1 T-sign on ocular B-scan ultrasound, denoting fluid in the sub-tenon space.

blood tests for aquaporin 4 and NMO antibodies should be considered if the neurological picture is very complicated.

Imaging: CT or MRI head and orbits should be considered for cases of orbital tumour, cranial nerve palsies, ocular ischaemic syndrome and optic neuritis. Carotid Doppler and FFA may also be indicated in ocular ischaemic syndrome, though the pain is usually through iris/angle neovascularisation, and this is for the most part self-evident.

DIAGNOSIS

Eye pain is an associated symptom. A detailed history and examination is prudent in forming a differential diagnosis. This will guide investigation, treatment and management. Not all investigations are necessary for all patients and should be guided on history and examination.

MANAGEMENT

Initial treatment is localised to the cause of pain, with investigation and subsequent management focused at controlling other associated factors. Time dependent emergencies will require the correct treatment to reduce the chances of irreparable damage to the eye.

Eyelids and face: Preseptal or orbital cellulitis will need antibiotics, orally, if preseptal, and IV if orbital. Admission and CT of the head is indicated in patients with orbital disease or who have no reduction in cellulitis despite 48 hours of oral antibiotics. Rapid release of retobulbar haemorrhage with canthotomy is essential, and and maxillofacial referral where fractures are found.

Anterior segment: Corneal infections and abrasions can be treated with topical antibiotics. Severe infections will need hourly treatment as per local guidelines. Consider admission in severe cases whereby hourly drops are needed. Topical antivirals are useful for herpetic disease. Cylcoplegics can be beneficial, though beware of a shallow anterior chamber that may tip the patient into an attack of angle closure glaucoma.

Raised IOP: Acute angle glaucoma is treated with topical pilocarpine, predforte, timolol and IV and/or oral acetazolamide. The aim of treatment is to break the cycle in which the acute angle attack has happened. Iridotomies and/or cataract surgery will be needed as long-term treatment for these patients. Beware of differentials including phacomorphic glaucoma and aqueous misdirection where the management needs to be tailored. Neovascular glaucoma should be managed IOP medically, then urgent PRP is required with dilated examination and consideration of cyclodiode on glaucoma review.

Medical referral: Cranial nerve palsies associated with pain, optic neuritis or ocular ischaemia need further investigation and referral to a medical team for further investigation, including imaging and bloods. Temporal tenderness should be investigated as GCA and discussed with rheumatology.

FOLLOW UP

Mild: Patients presenting with simple ocular surface disease, conjunctivitis or mild preseptal cellulitis can be discharged with advice and treatment.

Moderate: Corneal infections need to be reviewed every other day, for 1–2 weeks depending on severity; with treatment, small dot infiltrates can be reviewed in a week. Uveitis can be reviewed 1–2 weeks after starting treatment and depending on progress may need further review and treatment.

Severe: Acute angle glaucoma needs to be reviewed weeks to months after definitive treatment has been initiated and IOP stabilised, to ensure the pressure is still under control. Beware the mixed mechanism!

General: Cranial nerve palsies, optic neuritis and ocular ischaemia need to be reviewed in general/neuro-ophthalmology or MR clinics as appropriate, weeks to months after initial investigations and referrals have been made to the relevant medical teams.

Inform patients to return to the urgent eye care service if symptoms get worse, as at times ocular signs may manifest a few days after the initial symptoms, or the treatment is not doing its job and needs to be reviewed.

PITFALLS

1. This biggest pitfall is not gaining enough information from the referring party, which may cause unnecessary delays. Eye pain is a symptom that can be either nothing, or something potentially sight-threatening and if the referrer is unsure of things and generally vague it is better to see the patient to be on the safe side. Eye pain is distressing and we should have a low threshold to see patients being referred for this.
2. Another common pitfall is not measuring and documenting corneal defects, hypopyon, hyphaema, or marking areas of cellulitis. It is a simple thing to do and a definitive way to determine if the infection or inflammation is improving. Consider photography as well.
3. Following up with non-responding patients in eye casualty for too long, possibly by passing them on to different trainees, who have never seen them before, is bad medicine. Do not avoid your responsibility to the patient. Do what needs to be done and don't dump on others; it is bad for the patient and bad for others. Instead, get sub-specialty input as soon as you can.

FURTHER READING

Denniston A., P. Murray. *The Oxford Handbook of Ophthalmology*. Oxford University Press, 2009.

Friedberg M., C. Rapuano. *The Wills Eye Manual*. LWW, 2012.

Williams G. S., M. Westcott. *Practical Uveitis: Understanding the Grape*. Taylor & Francis Group, 2017.

16 Retinal Tears and Detachments

Sidath Wijetilleka

KEY POINTS

1. Retinal tears and detachments can be blinding conditions if not treated promptly
2. Patients require a full dilated eye examination of both eyes
3. The presence of tobacco dust is an indicator of a retinal break

DIAGRAM OF ALGORITHM

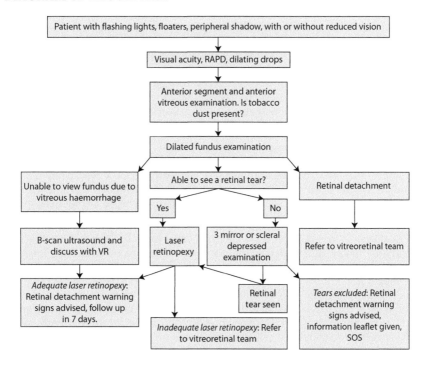

REFERRAL AND PRESENTATION

The most common presentation involves a new onset of floaters. The patient may describe seeing 'tadpoles', black dots or 'flies' for example. These tadpoles may be associated with flashing lights (Moore's lightning streak) which are more noticeable in the temporal aspect of their vision and as they go from bright to dim lighting. Patients often complain of chronic floaters but usually in a change of posterior segment anatomy this will be accompanied by a new onset of floaters differentiating them from everyday regular floaters. A complaint of a persistent shadow or dark curtain in the vision with peripheral or central vision loss is a sign of more serious retinal pathology that will require a thorough examination. Patients usually present to their optometrist with these typical symptoms, however, if out of regular working hours they may well present to A&E with a complaint of flashing lights and floaters or loss of vision. Risk factors for developing retinal tears include high myopia, trauma, pseudophakia, aphakia, previous retinal tears or detachments, family history and collagen disorders and peripheral retinal degeneration types.

DIFFERENTIAL DIAGNOSIS

Retinal tear ± vitreous haemorrhage: Retinal tears can take many form including, horse shoe U-shaped tears, linear tears or round holes. With U-shaped tears, the risk of detachment is high as often vitreous is still attached causing traction. Therefore, the risk of detachment is lower with operculated holes. Dark pigmentary changes around a tear or hole signifies chronicity suggesting it may have been there for some time. The flap of a tear is often still attached to the vitreous causing traction on the tear. Through the centre of the tear the underlying orange glow of the choroid can be visible.

Haemorrhagic or non-haemorrhagic posterior vitreous detachment: A posterior vitreous detachment (PVD) can elicit similar symptoms to a retinal tear. If the posterior hyaloid face detaches from a retinal vessel it may cause a release of blood into the pre-retinal space. This is known as a haemorrhagic PVD. Depending on the extent and density of the haemorrhage the view of the fundus may be obscured. In mild to moderate cases the peripheral retina can be visualised and peripheral retinal tears excluded. A complete vitreous haemorrhage in a patient without proliferative diabetic retinopathy warrants further investigation with a B-scan with prompt VR referral for potential surgical intervention.

Diabetic vitreous haemorrhage: In patients with proliferative diabetic retinopathy new blood vessels are formed which are prone to bleeding. They can bleed into the subhyaloid space causing a subhyaloid haemorrhage. Patients can have similar symptoms with floaters and a loss of vision if the haemorrhage is extensive. Usually a history of proliferative diabetic retinopathy with no retinal detachment on B-Scan ultrasound establishes the diagnosis.

Rhegmatogenous retinal detachment: Retinal detachments form once a tear has recruited enough fluid to detach the neurosensory retina surrounding it. In fact, the pressure generated by the RPE in holding down the neurosensory retina is less than 1 mm Hg so it does not take much force at all to tear the two layers of the retina apart. Retinal detachments appear as a cystic swelling of the retina often with a corrugated surface. The cyst appearance is due to the presence of underlying subretinal fluid. The presence of proliferative vitreoretinopathy (PVR) is demonstrated often by a whitish scar tissue on the retina or by stiff retinal folds which tend not to move with fluid vectors (see Figure 16.1). This is a sign of scar tissue formation, which leads to a poorer prognosis of retinal attachment.

Retinoschisis: This is derived from a microcystoid degeneration of the neurosensory retina with splitting at the level of the outer plexiform layer. Retinoschisis is more common in hyperopes and generally occurs inferiorly, temporally and commonly bilaterally. Myopic patients are much more likely to have retinal detachments than a retinoschisis. These can be differentiated through recognition that a retinoschisis causes an absolute scotoma whilst a detachment does not and that argon laser applied to the retina causes a visible burn in an area of retinoschisis but not with a detachment. There are also differences on examination though these are variable and should not be relied upon so will not be mentioned here.

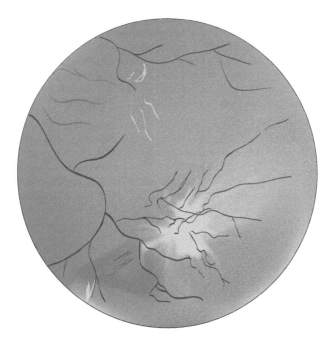

Figure 16.1 Proliferative vitreoretinopathy.

Non rhegmatogenous retinal detachments: This can be due to a range of diseases described below:

Inflammatory disease: Such as Vogt–Koyanagi–Harada (VKH) syndrome, posterior scleritis and other chronic inflammatory processes. This traditionally causes multiple serous detachments.

Neoplasia: Choroidal melanoma, metastasis, choroidal haemangioma, multiple myeloma, capillary retinal haemangioma can all present with exudative retinal detachments.

Congenital abnormalities: Optic pits, morning-glory syndrome and choroidal coloboma may also present with detachment of the neuro-sensory retina.

Vascular: Coats' disease and malignant hypertension both have exudative retinal detachments.

Ocular hypotension: Glaucoma drainage surgery may result in choroidal detachments which can mimic retinal detachments. If the choroidal detachments are not touching they can often resolve once the intraocular pressure has been re-established.

Other Causes of Pathological Floaters

Vitritis: It may well be difficult to differentiate pigmented anterior vitreous cells (tobacco dust) from either fine red blood cells or inflammatory vitreous cells. In vitritis the inflammatory cells are usually found in both the posterior and anterior chambers, and the cells are not typically pigmented. Vitritis tends to be a bilateral process with potentially but not always an underlying systemic disorder. Conventionally tobacco dust is a 'Y' shaped brown filament which is seen in the anterior vitreous. Fine red blood cells associated with vitreous haemorrhage can be associated with a retinal tear if a bridging vessel is involved which runs across the retinal break. Vitreous haemorrhages may also be a result of proliferative diabetic retinopathy or trauma; it is however imperative to rule out a retinal tear when faced with a vitreous haemorrhage and this is a golden rule.

Migraine: Flashing lights and zig zag patterns are perceived by patients suffering from migraines. The preceding aura associated with a migraine can often involve multi-coloured flashing lights and squiggly lines, which can obscure vision. Resolution of the flashing lights and visual obscuration once the migraine attack has subsided are classic signs of migraine aura. The key association of a headache and normal vitreous and retinal examination rule out retinal pathology and neurological causes should be excluded.

CLINICAL EXAMINATION

Visual acuity should be measured and documented. Check for the presence of a relative afferent pupillary defect (RAPD) to ascertain retinal function, especially in the case of an obstructed fundus examination. The presence of an RAPD could help indicate a cause of VH such as an ischaemic CRVO versus a peripheral retinal tear in an otherwise healthy eye.

Intraocular pressure: Should be measured, with Goldmann tonometry being the most reliable method in patients with potentially very high or low intraocular levels. Usually very bullous retinal detachments cause a reduction in intraocular pressure compared to the fellow eye.

Dilate: Any patient presenting with flashing lights and floaters warrants a dilated fundal examination of both eyes. The patient should be warned that their pupils may remain dilated for 4 to 6 hours and that they should not drive in this time.

Tobacco dust: After dilation the presence of tobacco dust (Shafer's sign) should be checked by shortening the beam to a 1×1 mm beam and obliquely shining it into the anterior vitreous. The patient should then be asked to look up and down and left to right to mobilise the vitreous. A positive finding of tobacco dust is often associated with release of retinal pigment epithelial cells suggesting a retinal break somewhere on the retina.

Lens: The lens status of the patient should be noted, as a poor view of the posterior segment due to cataract or potentially unstable IOL placement could have potential surgical implications. Document if the patient is pseudophakic and the location of the IOL ('in the bag' or 'in the sulcus').

Fundus: Dilated indirect ophthalmoscopy should be performed with a 90-diopter or widefield viewing lens. A thorough examination of the peripheral retina should be undertaken out to the ora serrata in search of retinal breaks. If this is not possible then a contact lens such as a three mirror lens should be used to visualise the peripheral retina out to the ora serrata.

Indentation: If a break is still not found then an indirect ophthalmoscopy using a 20 dioptre lens and 360° scleral indentation is used to view the peripheral retina. This is done by reclining the patient or laying them supine. The eye should receive topical anaesthesia and the patient warned that they may feel slight discomfort.

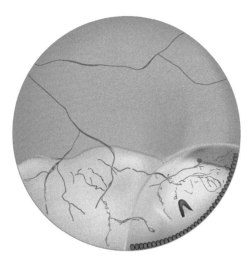

Figure 16.2 A peripheral retinal break visible on indentation with indirect ophthalmoscopy.

A Schocket depressor is used to gently depress the sclera and bring into view the peripheral retina to be checked for any tears (see Figure 16.2). If in doubt, seek senior advice or review.

INVESTIGATIONS

B-scan ultrasound: A B-scan should be performed when fundal view is obscured, in order to establish the integrity of the retina and presence of breaks. The retina's firm adherence to the optic disc gives a clue to whether a retinal detachment or posterior vitreous detachment has occurred. If the retina is attached to the disc but a funnel shaped elevation occurs then there is a retinal detachment until proven otherwise. If there is a uniform separation from the optic disc then this is almost certain to be a posterior vitreous detachment. Looking for retinal breaks using ultrasound can be tricky, but any discontinuity in a retinal area where there is still attachment to the optic disc should be suspected to be a retinal tear. B-scan in these cases is a dynamic investigation, with the movement of a hyperechoic line studied to discern the difference between a PVD, haemorrhage or detachment.

Optical coherence tomography (OCT): OCT scans can be useful in delineating the retinal layers to confirm a retinoschisis or to exclude subretinal fluid and hence a retinal detachment. If you are unsure whether the macula is involved in a retinal detachment, then OCT scans of the scans are useful in confirming macular involvement.

DIAGNOSIS

The diagnosis of a retinal tear or detachment is a clinical one. Once the tear or detachment has been located it should be precisely documented and drawn in the notes. The extent of the detachment including involvement of the macula should be documented as well as any identification of any retinal breaks. The fellow eye should also be thoroughly examined to rule out any ocular pathology.

MANAGEMENT

Retinal tears: Tears not associated with significant subretinal fluid should undergo immediate argon laser retinopexy. Urgent VR referral should be made for giant retinal tears, those with multiple breaks, patients with Stickler's, children and those with vitreous haemorrhage.

Laser retinopexy:

- The patient should be consented for this and topical anaesthesia used.

- A quadraspheric contact lens or a 3 mirror lens can be placed on the eye and the patient be comfortably seated at the Argon or Pascal laser machine.

- Settings of 200 mw × 200 ms × 200 microns × 0.2 ms are used to place three confluent rows around the tear, increasing the power until white burns are seen. Patients should be warned to expect a little bit of pain lest they jump as the laser is applied.

  - The aim is to create a firm chorioretinal adhesion in the attached retina around the tear to prevent subretinal fluid extending into healthy attached retina.

  - The anterior aspect of the tear is crucial as by not applying adequate laser here, the tear and subretinal fluid can spread. If the laser retinopexy is inadequate then cryotherapy may be needed to freeze the tear.

Retinal detachments and dialyses: Those not involving the macula are treated as emergencies and usually undergo urgent surgery within 24 hours. This is to preserve the macular function of the eye, which has not yet been compromised by being involved in the area of detachment. If the macula is detached then the prognosis of regaining good visual function is already poor, and thus surgery can afford to wait more than 24 hours. The various ways of fixing detachments, with vitrectomy and gas or cryobuckle will not be discussed here as they are not the concern of the casualty officer, but can be volunteered if the patient asks, or if a flight is imminent.

FOLLOW UP

Retinal tears: An isolated retinal tear treated with adequate laser retinopexy should be followed up in 1 week time, ideally by yourself. If there are any concerns about incomplete laser around the tear the patient should be brought back for an urgent vitreoretinal opinion. If adequate laser has been applied and there are no signs of any new tears developing the patient can be discharged with written information about the warning signs of a retinal detachment. In many departments specific leaflets are provided for just this scenario. If there are multiple tears then the patient should be followed up for a further 2–4 weeks.

Retinal detachments: Patients undergoing surgery are followed up by the vitreoretinal team.

FURTHER READING

American Academy of Ophthalmology Retina/Vitreous Panel. *Preferred Practice Pattern Guidelines. Posterior Vitreous Detachment, Retina Breaks, and Lattice Degeneration.* San Francisco, CA: American Academy of Ophthalmology, 2014.

PITFALLS

1. The biggest pitfall is not performing a dilated fundus examination of both eyes.
2. The second is not identifying tobacco dust.
3. The third is not identifying a retinal break in the presence of tobacco dust.
4. Correct technique in viewing the peripheral retina with indirect ophthalmoscopy and scleral indentation requires practice to master.

17 One or More Bulging Eyes

Derek Kwun-hong Ho

KEY POINTS

1. Thyroid eye disease is the most common cause of both unilateral and bilateral proptosis in adults.
2. Many causes of proptosis are sight-threatening. Some are even life-threatening.
3. Exposure keratopathy and compressive optic neuropathy are serious complications of proptosis.
4. Patients with thyroid eye disease should be told the importance of smoking cessation.

DIAGRAM OF ALGORITHM

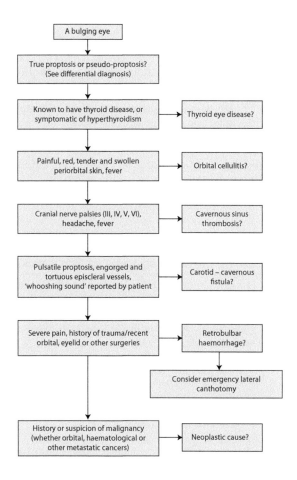

REFERRAL AND PRESENTATION

Proptosis, also sometimes called exophthalmos, is the abnormal axial or non-axial protrusion of the eyeball of which Thyroid eye disease (TED) is the most common cause in adults. As proptosis can be caused by a diverse range of local and systemic diseases, it is impossible to generalise the patient characteristics or source of referrals. They may be sent to you by the endocrinologist due to TED symptoms, or by the GP/optometrist for suspected periorbital cellulitis. They may be referred by the emergency department with a painful proptosed eye post-trauma or after orbital, lid or sinus surgery, for which retrobulbar haemorrhage must be ruled out.

Beware that the patient may present to you with other symptoms such as diplopia, reduced visual acuity, red eye, pain and grittiness and may not actually complain of proptosis at all. In such cases, the proptosis may have been overlooked by the patient or referring practitioner, or it may have been progressing slowly and the underlying disease taking a more insidious course.

As the exophthalmometer is typically only found in the ophthalmology department, it is highly unlikely that the referring source would contain more than a subjective remark of 'the eye looks proptosed'. It would, of course, be the eye casualty officer's task to try to quantify or refute this claim!

DIFFERENTIAL DIAGNOSIS

A wide range of local and systemic conditions can lead to proptosis (See Table 17.1). Therefore, it is helpful to use the 'surgical sieve' when considering the diverse differentials of unilateral and bilateral proptosis, such as VITAMIN (vascular, infective/inflammatory, traumatic, autoimmune, metabolic, idiopathic & neoplastic).

Thyroid eye disease (TED): is the most common cause of both unilateral and bilateral proptosis in adults. The average age of onset for TED is around 40 s and is more common in females. With 90% of TED patients suffering from Grave's disease (autoimmune hyperthyroidism), it is worth asking direct questions in associating hyperthyroid symptoms such as weight loss, palpitation, sweating and heat intolerance (your patient may indeed be wearing light clothing in cold weather). It is, however, important to note that some patients with sub-clinical disease do not develop symptoms of hyperthyroidism even after the onset of TED.

Table 17.1: **The Differential Diagnosis of Proptosis**

Vascular:	Carotid-cavernous fistula, cavernous haemangioma, orbital varix
Infective:	Orbital cellulitis, cavernous sinus thrombosis, mucomycosis, dacroadenitis
Inflammatory:	Thyroid eye disease, orbital inflammatory disease
Traumatic (including post-surgery):	Retrobulbar haemorrhage, globe displacement (see pseudo-proptosis below)
Autoimmune:	Orbital vasculitis (such as granulomatosis with polyangiitis, also known as Wegener's granulomatosis, polyarteritis nodosa)
Metabolic:	Cushing's syndrome
Idiopathic:	Idiopathic orbital inflammatory disease (also known as orbital pseudo-tumour – a diagnosis of exclusion!)
Neoplastic:	Orbital tumours (including lymphoma, glioma, meningioma, rhabdosarcoma, schwannoma), lacrimal gland tumour etc.

Beware of pseudo-proptosis, where the eye may appear to be protruding, when in fact it is the contralateral eye that is abnormal due to enophthalmos or ptosis, ipsilateral lid retraction with scleral show, buphthalmos, high axial length or facial asymmetry for example.

CLINICAL EXAMINATION

It is important to assess optic nerve function, including visual acuity, colour vision, pupillary reaction and visual field, which may guide the urgency and intensity of subsequent investigation and treatment.

Exophthalmometry: The exophthalmometer is used to measure axial proptosis. The make of the instrument should be documented (e.g. Keeler, Oculus) as they may give different horizontal width values even on the same patient. The difference between two eyes in a normal subject should be ≤ 2 mm. Upper limits are around 22 mm for Caucasians and 24 mm for Afro-Caribbeans. Beware that the accuracy of this test depends on symmetry of patient's lateral orbital rims which can be damaged by previous trauma, though the examiner's technique is by far the biggest variable!

Lids and orbit: Examine and palpate for mass or swelling in the eyelid, around the globe or behind the globe on retropulsion. Document mass features: site, size, surface/overlying skin, colour, contour, consistency, temperature, transillumination, tethering and tenderness to underlying structure. Palpate for swelling in the head and neck lymph nodes, which may point towards an infective or neoplastic cause, with temporal fullness for example being due to sphenoid wing meningioma.

Gentle palpation of the globe with your fingers may detect pulsatility and globe auscultation may reveal orbital bruit, which suggests a diagnosis of carotid-cavernous fistula (CCF), or rarely an AV malformation; this is one of the rare instances when stethoscopes are used in clinical ophthalmology. Proptosis that worsens with Valsalva manoeuvre and face down posturing suggests an orbital varix.

Ocular motility: Should be examined, which may reveal mechanical restriction in eye movement or involvement of other cranial nerves. Examining ductions, versions, a force duction test or performing a Hess chart will help to differentiate a mechanical versus neurological cause of restriction. A formal orthoptist report should be obtained.

Document the amount of superior and inferior scleral show, the presence of ptosis, lagophthalmos, Bell's phenomenon and corneal sensation. Observe their natural blinking motion (i.e. whether there is blink lagophthalmos).

Anterior segment: A painless, 'fleshy' salmon-pink patch on the conjunctiva can be a sign of conjunctival lymphoma. Engorged and tortuous episcleral vessels, on the other hand, may be caused by elevated venous pressure in the orbit. Look for signs of corneal exposure and ulceration with the aid of fluorescein.

Intraocular pressure (IOP): Intraocular pressure check is mandatory as the proptosed eye may be hypertensive due to pressure on the globe and require topical treatment (or even surgical in the case of retrobulbar haemorrhage). IOP rise during up gaze is exaggerated in TED due to inferior rectus muscle enlargement.

Optic disc: Appearance should be documented for swelling, pallor, venous congestion and the presence of spontaneous venous pulsation. Comparisons should be made especially in unilateral proptosis cases. Visual fields can be used to document any optic neuropathy.

Table 17.2: The Clinical Activity Score (CAS)

Pain	1. Spontaneous retrobulbar ache
	2. Pain on attempted up, lateral or down gaze
Redness	3. Redness of the eyelids
	4. Redness of the conjunctiva
Swelling	5. Swelling of the eyelids
	6. Inflammation of the caruncle and/or plica
	7. Conjunctival oedema (chemosis)

Source: Modified from Mourits M. P. et al. *British Journal of Ophthalmology*, 73(8): 1989; 639–644.
Note: A CAS of ≥3 indicates active disease.

Put together your examination findings to give a clinical activity score (CAS – See Table 17.2), which measures the classical features of inflammation in TED (pain, redness and swelling). A CAS of ≥3 (out of 7) indicates active disease.

Where possible arrange clinical photographs of the patient's face and eye position/proptosis. This may be impossible if seeing the patient out of hours, but the patient can take them on their smartphone.

INVESTIGATIONS

Bloods: As TED is the most common cause, blood based investigation for thyroid function and thyroid simulating immunoglobulin is mandatory in most cases of proptosis. FBC and inflammatory markers may also be deranged in haematological malignancies and infective causes. An autoimmune screen for vasculitic causes of proptosis may also be performed, including ESR, CRP, FBC, glucose and cANCA. Specific tests for IgG4 may be requested where orbital inflammatory conditions are suspected.

Imaging: Urgent computer tomography (CT) or magnetic resonance imaging (MRI) would also be indicated if there is some doubt as to the cause, and especially if there is suspicion of optic nerve compromise. It is important to request an 'orbital scan' so detailed fine cuts are taken through the orbit and clearly document what pathology you suspect so the radiologists can perform the most suitable imaging. The normal intraorbital segment of the optic nerve has an average 6 mm of slack, seen as a gentle curvature on imaging, meaning that there is small amount of potential room for the globe to proptose without the optic nerve being stretched.

- Contrast will help the reporting radiologist detect vascular causes of proptosis more easily.

- Neuroimaging with STIR sequence MRI in TED may show fusiform enlargement of extraocular muscles, commonly affecting the inferior and medial recti with sparing of muscle tendons (see Figure 17.1).

- Neuroimaging has the additional benefit of objectively quantifying the amount of proptosis, without the inherent parallax error and inter-observer difference from exophthalmometry, though there are ophthalmologists out there who claim that their measurement of proptosis is indeed superior to that of formal imaging.

Very occasionally, orbital biopsy is required for a histological diagnosis if the above investigations have not yet yielded a diagnosis, though such cases would be under the care of an oculoplastics specialist by then.

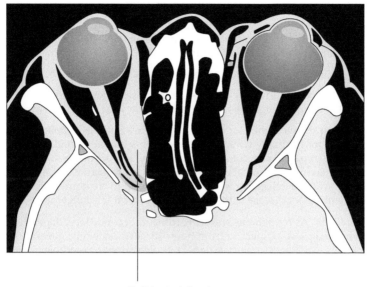

Medial rectus belly enlargement

Figure 17.1 Axial CT orbit of a patient with TED, showing bilateral proptosis and (most prominently) medial recti muscle belly enlargement. Note the narrow tendinous insertions in contrast.

DIAGNOSIS

As above, proptosis is a clinical sign for which there are many possible causes. Once an underlying diagnosis is made, referral to the relevant medical, radiological or surgical specialties should be sent promptly.

MANAGEMENT

Supportive management may involve intensive ocular lubricants by day and ointment overnight. In cases of corneal exposure, consider botulinum toxin injections to reduce upper lid retraction and induce ptosis or temporary tarsorrhaphy may be required to reduce the risk of corneal ulceration or perforation (see Chapter 6). When faced with ulceration or perforation IOP lowering treatment should be commenced where needed. Disease specific treatments are discussed below.

Retrobulbar haemorrhage: Early diagnosis and perform an emergency lateral canthotomy and inferior cantholysis to relieve orbital compression and monitor optic nerve function.

Thyroid eye disease: In sight-threatening dysthyroid optic neuropathy (DON):

- Systemic glucocorticoid use such as pulsed intravenous methyl-prednisolone (IVMP) may be indicated – liaise with senior colleagues and rule out contraindications.

- Concurrent bone protection medications should be given.

- Close monitoring of blood pressure and blood sugar is also required as high dose steroid use can destabilise these parameters.

- Patients may then be given a course of oral steroids after the IVMP treatment.

- Orbital radiotherapy and orbital decompression surgery may also be considered; these should be guided by the oculoplastic specialist's expertise and depends on local availability.

- Selenium supplementation has also been shown to be beneficial.

- Finally, one should always discuss smoking cessation (and document it) with TED patients; though this is not traditionally your concern in eye casualty.

Beware that the more sinister causes of proptosis such as lymphoma and other malignancies may initially respond somewhat to systemic steroid with shrinkage and therefore apparent clinical improvement, though of course masking the true disease and making subsequent biopsy and histological diagnosis more challenging. This is of particular relevance when steroid is used to treat presumed idiopathic orbital inflammatory disease without excluding other more dangerous differentials.

Other conditions: As for patients suffering from other conditions, depending on the underlying diagnosis, expertise from neurosurgery, oncology, general medicine, microbiology, paediatrics, interventional radiology or neuro-radiology teams may need to be called upon. The role of an eye casualty officer in such cases will be to ensure that the patient's visual function is regularly assessed and the under-moisturised ocular surface is looked after, whether as an inpatient or outpatient.

See Chapter 2 for management of orbital cellulitis.

FOLLOW UP

Frequency of follow-up should be tailored to the perceived risks to the patient's visual function and state of the ocular surface in your orbital or oculoplastic clinics. Patients should be reminded to re-attend urgently to the eye casualty in the event of any symptoms of corneal disease or optic nerve compromise.

Thyroid eye disease: Patients should be followed up in an oculoplastics, TED specialist clinic with orthoptic input. Surgical treatment for proptosis in TED occurs in a very specific order: orbital decompression, strabismus correction then eyelid repositioning. Eventually patients will reach a 'burn-out' stage, when the disease activity has quieted and TED features have stabilised lowering the risk of visual loss.

PITFALLS

1. Not measuring the amount of proptosis with an exophthalmometer. Try to use the same make of instrument and the same horizontal width value consistently in follow-up appointments, for more reliable comparison and to better track the patient's progress.
2. Not arranging suitable follow up to monitor for changes in visual function or informing the patient to return quickly if they experience problems.
3. It may also be easy to forget about managing the dry eye while the more 'exciting' tasks such as making phone calls to other departments to arrange imaging or admission take place. This should be considered as a task exclusive to ophthalmologists; an inpatient with dementia who has severe dry eye but cannot verbalise their ocular pain can develop corneal perforation, or a red gritty eye may be treated by other doctors on the ward with preserved chloramphenicol eye drops as a 'lubricant' for months.

FURTHER READING

Bartalena, L. et al. Consensus statement of the European Group on Graves' Orbitopathy (EUGOGO) on management of GO. *European Journal of Endocrinology*, 158(3): 2008; 273–285.

Calvano, C. J. *Smith and Nesi's Ophthalmic Plastic and Reconstructive Surgery.* Springer Science & Business Media, 2012.

Mourits M. P., Koornneef L., Wiersinga W. M., Prummel M. F., Berghout A., van der Gaag R. Clinical criteria for the assessment of disease activity in Graves' ophthalmopathy: A novel approach. *British Journal of Ophthalmology*, 73(8): 1989; 639–644.

18 Double Vision and New Onset Strabismus in an Adult

Eulee Seow

KEY POINTS

1. Check what the patient means by double vision – is it monocular or binocular?
2. History and speed of onset can give an indication of underlying causes
3. Organise urgent imaging in pupil involving third nerve palsies or sixth nerve palsies with papilloedema
4. Warn patients with sudden onset double vision not to drive
5. Always rule out GCA

DIAGRAM OF ALGORITHM

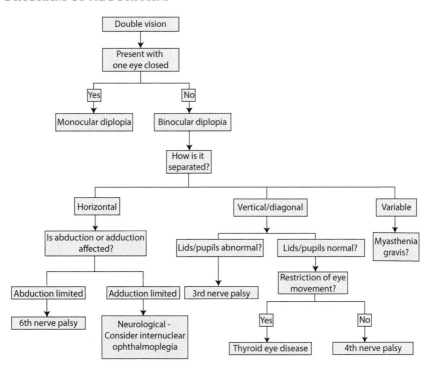

REFERRAL AND PRESENTATION

Patients usually present with blurred vision or double vision, termed diplopia. Check what they mean by double vision, and also check if it is monocular or binocular by covering each eye in turn. If the double vision persists with an eye covered then it is defined as monocular diplopia and the cause lies within that eye and its refractive media rather than being a fault of ocular motility. An orthoptist will not be interested in monocular diplopia.

123

For binocular double vision, history taking is targeted at first identifying the potential causes, whether the problem is vascular or restrictive for example, and identifying the ocular motility deficit. There are four aspects to consider: the speed of onset, direction of the double vision, associated features and past medical history of note.

Firstly let us consider the speed of onset. Ask when the patient first noticed it, what were they doing at the time, if it has changed, if it varies through the day, and if they are still noticing it. A history of sudden onset suggests a vascular cause, while a fluctuating onset can indicate decompensation of a neuromuscular cause. A slowly worsening double vision can either represent a mechanical or restrictive issue.

Secondly, ask about the direction of double vision. Ask if the double vision is vertical, horizontal or diagonal and if it changes with the position of gaze. Identify the direction of gaze and when the separation of images is at its worst. This can help with identifying the motility deficit.

Thirdly, identify any associated features such as headaches, ptosis, eye pain, previous trauma and head posture.

Lastly, ask about past medical history. Specifically ask about a history of previous squint/lazy eye/ patching as a child, any previous surgery to the eye or any recent trauma. Also enquire about vascular risk factors such as diabetes or previous strokes.

DIFFERENTIAL DIAGNOSIS

Using the above four-step algorithm one can come up with a probable list of differential diagnoses for binocular diplopia prior to examining the patient, (remember VITAMIN as your surgical sieve).

Vascular: Patients with vascular causes of diplopia either have the microvasculature to blame secondary to diabetes and hypertension or an aneurysm pressing on the nerve, which traditionally causes a third nerve palsy.

Inflammatory: Such causes of diplopia can be secondary to thyroid eye disease, orbital myositis, or neuroinflammatory disorders, which can cause an internuclear ophthalmoplegia for example, and tends to be fairly constant.

Traumatic: This mainly consists of diplopia secondary to an orbital floor fracture and eye movement is painful and highly restrictive in the affected eye. The history is obvious here.

Neuro-muscular: Myasthenia gravis is a problem at the neuromuscular junction that classically causes fatigability with diplopia being very variable and worse toward the end of the day.

Infective: Orbital cellulitis, which at its worst could cause an orbital apex syndrome, can cause diplopia though the wealth of other symptoms and usually makes this a secondary consideration.

Tumours: These can be either orbital or intracranial and cause restrictive diplopia if in the orbit or cause neural issues if intracranial.

Decompensation: The delicate balancing act yoking both eyes together can be upset by close work, by stress, by coffee and a host of other issues and cause a variable diplopia.

CLINICAL EXAMINATION

Examination will help localise the problem.

Afferent and efferent pathways: Assess the different systems separately, beginning with the afferent. Assess optic nerve function by recording the patient's visual acuity, colour vision, pupil reactions and fundoscopy. Consider confrontation or formal visual fields.

Monocular diplopia: Careful ophthalmic examination should reveal the cause of the double vision but generally symptoms improve with a pinhole. Causes include refractive error, astigmatism, an unstable tear film, cataract, post iridotomy or with a dislocated intraocular lens, for example.

Binocular diplopia: Observe the patient for an abnormal head posture (head tilt in a fourth nerve palsy and head turn in a sixth nerve palsy, or chin up in TED).

Saccades: Start the examination itself with an assessment of saccades, both horizontally and vertically. Slow saccades can occur in conditions such as neuropathy, myopathy or neuromuscular junction disorders such as myasthenia. Saccades are normally preserved in restrictive conditions, post trauma or thyroid eye disease. Some practitioners assess saccades after the main examination but the one true constant with assessment of ocular motility is that the majority of people do things slightly differently, with no evidence whatsoever that one method is superior to another.

The cover/uncover test: The cover/uncover test can reveal tropias while the alternate cover test reveals full tropias and latent phorias. This can be measured with prisms (apex towards deviation, i.e. base in for exotropia for example). Check eye movements (pursuit) of the eyes individually (ductions) and together (versions) in the nine positions of gaze (see Figure 18.1). Ocular alignment in the nine positions of gaze should be evaluated for distance and near.

Nystagmus: Look for rapid involuntary movements of the eyes and record their direction (horizontal/vertical/rotatory), amplitude and frequency.

Cranial nerves: Examine for involvement of other cranial nerves where appropriate via facial and corneal sensation (fifth cranial nerve), eyelid position and orbicularis strength.

Perform related examinations to help locate the problem, for example an orbital exam, including exophthalmometry for orbital apex pathology, or listening for a bruit for carotid cavernous sinus fistula. This is almost never detected properly by an ophthalmologist but comes up in exams.

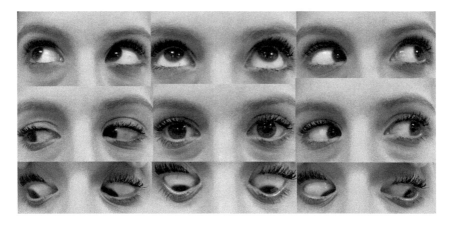

Figure 18.1   The nine positions of gaze.

INVESTIGATIONS

Investigations should be targeted using the clinical history and examination findings.

- An orthoptic assessment with measurements of angle of deviation and prism fusion range is useful in identifying the cause of binocular diplopia and treatment with prisms.

- *Bloods*: Consider assessment for vascular or inflammatory risk factors including BP, FBC, ESR, CRP, glucose and lipids to help rule out hypertension, diabetes or giant cell arteritis (GCA).

Other specific tests include:

Variable signs and symptoms of fatigue: Bloods to include serum autoantibodies (anti-acetylcholine receptor and anti-MUSK) for myasthenia gravis. The ice pack test: measure deviation or ptosis before and after applying an ice pack to the eyes for 2 minutes. However, in practice it is almost impossible to find ice in a regular eye clinic.

Proptosis, lid lag: Consider thyroid function, thyroid peroxidase and imaging for thyroid eye disease.

Imaging: MRI gives better soft tissue definition but CTs may be easier and faster to organise. Imaging will help identify bleeds, stroke, space occupying lesions, abnormal muscle size and vascular anomalies such as an aneurysm or carotid cavernous fistula.

DIAGNOSIS

Isolated third nerve palsy: The third cranial nerve innervates the superior rectus, medial rectus, inferior oblique and inferior rectus, the levator palpebrae superioris, pupillary sphincter and ciliary muscle pupillary fibres. Abnormality of the third nerve can occur at any point involving one or more branches. Palsy can cause a partial or complete ptosis with a 'down and out' eye (depressed and exotropic). Check for pupillary involvement; if the pupil is dilated and poorly responsive to light and accommodation an urgent scan is needed to exclude a posterior communicating artery aneurysm. A pupil involving complete third nerve palsy tends to be much more likely to be due to an aneurysm due to the superficial nature of the pupillary fibres whilst an incomplete pupil sparing third nerve palsy is more likely to be microvascular as the affected vasa nervorum disproportionately supplies the inside of the nerve and not the surface fibres.

Isolated sixth nerve palsy: The sixth cranial nerve innervates the lateral rectus. Patients complain of horizontal diplopia worse in the distance, and examination reveals a small esotropia with reduced abduction. Microvascular causes are common in older populations. In all, however, it is important to check for any signs of papilloedema to exclude a false localising sign of raised intracranial pressure.

Isolated fourth nerve palsy: A fourth cranial nerve palsy results in poor superior oblique function. Patients present with a contralateral head tilt and report vertical, oblique or torsional diplopia, worse on down gaze. Cover test shows an ipsilateral hypertropia worse on gaze to the contralateral side and ipsilateral head tilt. Fundoscopy may show excyclotorsion of ipsilateral eye which is apparent only when assessing the position of the arcades relative to the optic disc. Causes include head trauma (which may be bilateral), myasthenia gravis and thyroid eye disease. Decompensating congenital fourth nerve palsy can present with intermittent diplopia and old photographs may show a head tilt. This is colloquially called a 'family album tomogram'.

Multiple cranial nerve palsies: Orbital apex syndrome can occur due to inflammation or infection in the orbital apex or cavernous sinus. Patients can present with a combination of third, fourth and sixth nerve palsies with retro-orbital pain, conjunctival infection and possible facial numbness (fifth cranial involvement). Request urgent imaging, (preferably MRI), for these patients.

Myasthenia gravis (MG): Myasthenia gravis is a great mimicker and can result in variable diplopia and odd ocular motility patterns. It should be remembered as a differential diagnosis especially in the context of fluctuating symptoms. If a diagnosis of MG is established, a chest CT should be performed to rule out a thymoma, which occurs in about 10% of patients with MG.

Thyroid eye disease (TED): Thyroid eye disease can present with slowly progressive binocular diplopia, and is often worse in the morning. The inferior rectus is most commonly affected, followed by medial, superior and lateral recti and patients can present with vertical diplopia and a chin up position. Other findings include eyelid retraction or oedema, proptosis, positive forced ductions, and lagophthalmos. If suspected request thyroid function test, which is normal in up to 10% of patients, and anti thyroidperoxidase antibody. Orbital imaging can show enlargement of the extraocular muscles with sparing of the tendinous insertion (best seen on MRI). Advise patients to quit smoking if relevant.

Orbital trauma: Orbital trauma results in a mechanical restriction and will hopefully be evident in the history. Retrobulbar haemorrhage, fractures and muscle injury or entrapment can cause restriction in eye movement and diplopia. Maxillofacial teams like to confirm that the globe and optic nerve are intact so ensure that this is clearly recorded. They often ask for Hess charts for surgical planning, and it is important to accommodate this request in a timely manner.

Orbital cellulitis: Orbital cellulitis should be evident from the clinical examination, with lid swelling, redness and chemosis. If there is restriction of ocular motility check that the optic nerve is not compromised, organise an urgent scan to exclude a subperiosteal abscess, and refer to ENT. Differentials here include tumour and hypersensitivity reaction.

MANAGEMENT

Treatment of inflammatory, infectious and traumatic causes for diplopia will aim to improve symptoms according to aetiology.

Symptoms of diplopia: Offer occlusion to patients with symptomatic diplopia to ease discomfort. Prism (Fresnel) may be helpful in comitant deviations, and especially if there is diplopia in primary position. Advise patients with sudden onset diplopia not to drive (as per DVLA guidance).

FOLLOW UP

Arrange review with the relevant subspecialty for further follow up and orthoptist review.

- In patients with pain and pupil involving third nerve palsies request an urgent CTA/MRA to rule out an aneurysm.
- Refer atypical cranial nerve palsies for further investigation with medical/ neurological colleagues, i.e. those associated with multiple cranial nerves,

headaches, papilloedema or GCA symptoms. Neuro-ophthalmology review can be arranged, priority to those with optic nerve compromise.

- All other cranial nerve palsies without other neurological signs or symptoms; optimise cardiovascular risk factors. These patients can be monitored by the orthoptic team. If there is no recovery by 3 months further investigations such as imaging may be needed.

- In patients with suspected myasthenia gravis check that there is no pulmonary involvement; if so urgent referral to the medical team is needed. Refer to neurology for consideration of steroids or pyridostygmine following diagnosis.

- In thyroid eye disease check that there is no exposure and no acute optic neuropathy; if so high dose steroids may be needed and urgent orbital/ oculoplastic review should be arranged.

PITFALLS

1. In a patient with sixth nerve palsy always check for papilloedema as it could be a false localising sign for raised intracranial pressure.
2. Be sure to check FBC, ESR and CRP in an older patient to exclude GCA.
3. Pupil involving third nerve palsy cases require urgent CT head ±CT angiogram to rule out an aneurysm.
4. Check for involvement of other cranial nerves, especially facial and corneal sensation.
5. Warn patients not to drive if they are suffering from acute diplopia, and document that you have done so!

---

19 My Baby Has a White Pupil in This Photograph and/or Has a Squint

Ryan Davies

KEY POINTS

1. Most causes of leukocoria are sight/life threatening and therefore need urgent assessment
2. Take a detailed history
3. Do not dilate the child on arrival. Assess the optic nerve function and the anterior segment first
4. Fundal examination and baseline (gross) refraction is essential in all cases
5. B-scan is useful in difficult cases

DIAGRAM OF ALGORITHM: STRABISMUS/LEUKOCORIA

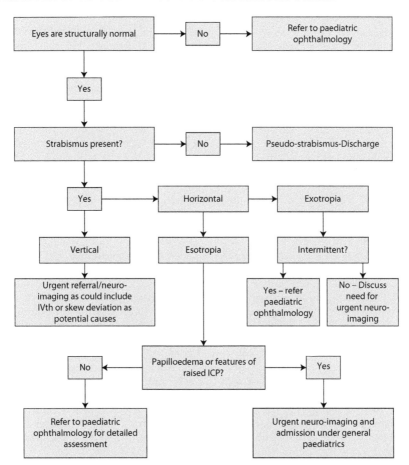

DIAGRAM OF ALGORITHM: NYSTAGMUS

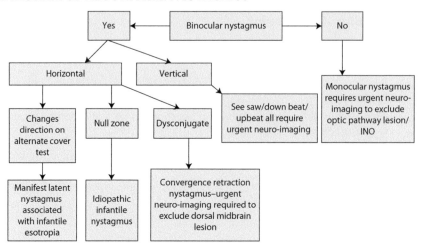

REFERRAL AND PRESENTATION

A child referred to a busy eye casualty department, particularly an infant, and particularly if they have a squint will broadly split trainee ophthalmologists into two categories. The first group will be reaching into their bag for their prism bars with eager anticipation of the patient's arrival, whereas the second group will be slightly more hesitant and suggest that an orthoptic assessment might be the better first port of call. Now of course the first group doesn't really exist, and in most cases the second group would be correct in requesting a detailed orthoptic assessment. Part of the reason for hesitancy is, of course, through no fault of their own lack of experience. The rest of the reason is the result of fear and trepidation in not wanting to miss a diagnosis that could be potentially blinding, or even worse, fatal for the child. It is therefore important to note early on in this chapter that an urgent referral for a child with a suspicious squint, abnormal eye movement or leukocoria, should not be delayed until an orthoptic appointment is made available. The initial assessment should be in the emergency department, in combination with or followed up by an orthoptic and/or paediatric ophthalmology assessment if necessary.

The presentation and source of referral can vary. All children in the UK should undergo screening at birth, at 6–8 weeks of life and then early on in their school years. A significant amount of referrals will therefore arise from 'abnormalities' detected during these assessments, and a large proportion of those will work their way directly into a paediatric ophthalmology clinic through established pathways. The remainder will result from in hospital referrals, optometrists or parental concern. Parents spend an awful lot of time looking at and comparing their children, and therefore any concerns raised should not be taken lightly. Whether it be the first time overly anxious father that wants reassurance that Sienna is normal, or the mother with five other children that says little Joey isn't behaving visually like his siblings did at the corresponding age. Finally we must pay a notable mention to rise of photographic ease, which comes with owning a smartphone. On average a parent will have between 10 to 15,000 images of their newborn on their camera phone, and as such we should expect an exponential increase in the number of 'abnormal' pupil reflexes detected.

DIFFERENTIAL DIAGNOSIS

The causes of squint and leukocoria will be considered separately here but it is important to note that there is a significant overlap, particularly if the cause of leukocoria results in a sensory deprivation amblyopia. For that reason, fundal examination is essential in all infants presenting with an abnormality of ocular alignment.

Leukocoria: Refers to an abnormal white appearance to the pupillary area (see Figure 19.1). In reality, referrals may not necessarily be due to leukocoria, but due to an absent or difference in the red reflex appearance between each eye. An absent red reflex, or reduced red reflex (whether they be white or not) also needs to be seen to exclude a potential treatable cause.

The most worrying cause of leukocoria and the one not to miss is retinoblastoma. If detected early, the eye, if not sight can be preserved. A late presentation unfortunately carries a significant mortality rate. For leukocoria to be present, one would expect a large, posterior retinoblastoma to be present and therefore within the capabilities of most trainee ophthalmologists to detect. Other causes can include but are not limited to cataract, Coats disease (significant exudation), toxocara, Coloboma and Norrie disease (retinal detachment). All causes of leukocoria are potentially sight threatening and therefore prompt referral and assessment is vital. In this author's experience, the common reasons for referral of absent red reflex is due to increased retinal pigmentation in Asian and Afro-Caribbean racial group individuals or a suspected abnormal pupil reflex may be raised by the parent after review of their children in photographs.

Strabismus: The main challenge with strabismus in an emergency department is identifying those that are caused by conditions that may need urgent investigation and onward referral. The remainder can be followed up in a paediatric clinic. The first question is whether this is a structurally normal eye. The next question is whether strabismus is present. Pseudo-strabismus is a common referral into eye departments. If strabismus is present then is it horizontal (esotropia or exotropia), vertical, torsional or a combination? Esotropias can be infantile, accommodative, neurological (secondary to sixth nerve palsy), sensory or due to a congenital cranial nerve dis-innervation disorder. A gross refraction and fundal examination are necessary in all cases, as not to miss the under corrected hypermetrope, or the

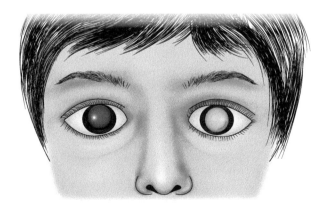

Figure 19.1   A child with leukocoria.

child with raging papilloedema. Exotropias can also be infantile, intermittent, constant, neurological and sensory. A constant exotropia in an infant is more suggestive of an underlying neurological cause and therefore has a low threshold for neuro-imaging. Associated movements such as nystagmus can also shed light on the underlying cause. A nystagmus that changes direction on alternate cover test is reassuring, where as a monocular or vertical nystagmus may need urgent investigation.

CLINICAL EXAMINATION

Your examination begins by observing the child in the waiting area: are they disproportionately distressed or overly sedated? How do they behave on entering the consultation room? Are there any obvious dysmorphic features? A basic knowledge of developmental milestones and visual development in children is therefore essential to identify a developmentally delayed child.

It is a cliché but a detailed clinical history is essential including presenting complaint, past medical history, drug history, vaccination history, maternal obstetric history and family history. Don't be afraid to utilise parental smartphone evidence. They will be all too happy to show you the extensive number of photographs that they have available with a clear timeline. Often, the squint that they are concerned about in a photo will show a child with equal corneal reflexes from the camera flash and a slight head turn away from the camera with prominent epicanthic folds or wide bridge to the nose.

If you are fortunate enough to have an orthoptist available then, of course, an assessment from them will provide a significant amount of information. If there is not one available then try your best to get a visual acuity. Again, knowledge of visual development and appropriate testing depending on the age of the child is essential. Are they fixing and following? Are they making good eye contact? Are they reaching for toys? Or are they not displaying reliable visual responses with roving eye movements. A detailed orthoptic examination will include assessment of visual, sensory and motor function. The extensive battery of tests that they can perform is not necessary in an emergency setting but assessment of vision and extra-ocular muscle movement is necessary. Look at the corneal reflexes, do a quick cover test and alternate cover test if nothing else. You won't have much time and may only get one shot at it. If there is a vertical deviation try to do the Bielschowsky 3-step test. If the vertical deviation significantly improves on lying the patient flat then this is suggestive of a skew deviation and neurological imaging is required.

If you are seeing the child for the first time always perform an assessment of optic nerve function as thoroughly as you can depending on the age of the child. A RAPD check should be the bare minimum. Avoid the temptation to ask the nurse to administer dilating drops on arrival and always assess the anterior segment first. This may save time now, but you may miss something important. IOP assessment is now relatively simple in children with the advent of rebound tonometers such as the I-CARE and should be done as a baseline in most cases.

A dilated examination is essential in all children presenting for the first time to an emergency department, especially if they have an abnormality of ocular alignment or abnormal pupil reflexes. If the child is younger than 6 months then cyclopentolate 0.5% ±phenylephrine 2.5% can be used and will provide adequate cycloplegia. If they are older than 6 months then cyclopentolate 1% can be used, or atropine 1% if they have particularly dark irises. Assess the red reflex for symmetry and uniformity. A nasal mass for example may have a normal red reflex if the child is looking to the opposite side. When assessing the phakic lens, always use a portable slit lamp where possible as lens opacities are not always necessarily evident with a red reflex check alone. The retinoscope is a useful tool as it often gives a clear red reflex even if the ophthalmoscope doesn't. Fundal examination is again essential in all cases. If you can't see or are not confident then don't be afraid to ask for a senior opinion, but practice makes perfect. A B-scan is always useful in the un-cooperative child with a difficult fundal view.

A quick cycloplegic refraction should be attempted. Do not split hairs about a 0.50D difference here and there; you just don't want to miss the child with a gross refractive error which needs treating and monitoring. There is no clinical relevance whatsoever to such minor differences in refraction.

INVESTIGATIONS

In the majority of cases a detailed orthoptic evaluation will be necessary. They will assess vision, sensory and motor function. It is important to be able to interpret orthoptic reports; ask your local friendly orthoptist to show you how to do so.

A B-scan ultrasound requires minimal compliance from the child. It will give an idea if there is a retinal detachment or a suspicious highly echogenic mass at the posterior pole. Depending on the age of the child an OCT scan can also provide a wealth of information.

A general Paediatric assessment may be necessary for a full assessment of the child to exclude any associated systemic abnormalities, especially if specific syndromes are suspected.

If there is a potential underlying neurological abnormality then neuro-imaging will be required, CT or MRI, usually led by the paediatricians as general anaesthesia may be required.

DIAGNOSIS

From an emergency ophthalmology perspective, the main aim is to identify whether an abnormality is actually present. Onward referral to general paediatrics and/or paediatric ophthalmology will then be necessary. The length of follow up will be dependent on the underlying abnormality; if in doubt discuss with a senior colleague.

MANAGEMENT

The management will depend on the underlying diagnosis. In an emergency setting the main aim is to exclude serious pathology. The follow up and future management will be in a paediatric ophthalmology clinic.

FOLLOW UP

The time to next follow up depends on the underlying cause. There are those cases where you need to physically march to the consultant to review your patient immediately, those that warrant an immediate phone call/fax/email and then those that warrant a routine dictated or typed referral.

Most causes of leukocoria can be sight threatening if not life threatening and therefore need to be seen by a specialist urgently. Retinoblastoma needs to be seen by a consultant immediately and referred on urgently to a specialist centre. Again, if you are not sure or not confident then ask for a senior opinion. This may avoid an unnecessary follow up at the very least. A congenital cataract for example would warrant a phone call discussion with a paediatric ophthalmologist with a special interest in paediatric cataract surgery to facilitate an urgent follow up appointment and plans for surgical intervention.

PITFALLS

1. Asking for an orthoptic assessment first can sometimes cause an unnecessary delay, depending on the availability in your unit. Delays are stressful for already anxious parents and also you will not get the necessary experience in assessing motility.
2. Avoid the temptation to save time by dilating the child on arrival. Exclude a RAPD and assess the red reflex when undilated. You may miss signs such as iris transillumination defects. Also, if there is a cataract present it is useful to know the extent obscuring the pupil when undilated.
3. Try to avoid documenting 'fundal view not possible' or 'unable to examine'. It will never be easy but if the child has had dilating drops, try your best to get most out of each assessment, even if it means asking for a senior opinion. Sending the family for a walk can calm both the child and stressed doctor, often resulting in the child falling asleep. A sleeping child is the ophthalmologist's best friend. Failing that, bribe with stickers. If everything else fails do a B-scan to potentially exclude a retinal detachment or calcified mass!

FURTHER READING

Lambert S., Lyons C. *Taylor and Hoyt's Pediatric Ophthalmology and Strabismus*, 5th edition, Elsevier, 2016.

20 Non-Accidental Injury

Damien Yeo

KEY POINTS
1. Retinal haemorrhages are part of the triad of shaken baby syndrome (retinal haemorrhages, subdural haematoma, and encephalopathy)
2. A negative finding is as important as a positive finding
3. The diagnosis has important medicolegal implications so documentation has to be detailed every step of the way
4. If possible, all retinal haemorrhages need to be photographed as early as possible

DIAGRAM OF ALGORITHM

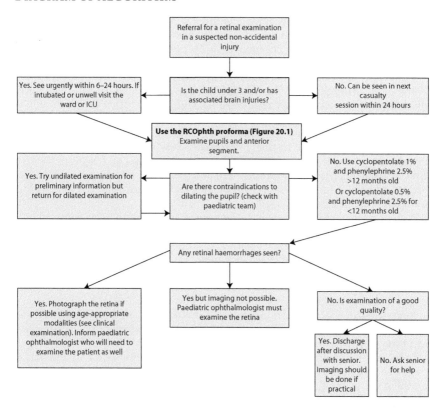

REFERRAL AND PRESENTATION
Virtually all non-accidental injury (NAI) referrals will come from the paediatricians, specifically the child protection team. In cases of paediatric head trauma where NAI is suspected as a differential diagnosis the paediatricians are interested in the

135

presence/absence of retinal haemorrhages. Retinal haemorrhages are a relevant finding because they have a high positive predictive rate for abusive head trauma.

The terms non-accidental injury (NAI), non-accidental head injury (NAHI), shaken baby syndrome (SBS), and abusive head trauma (AHT) have been used interchangeably in the past. The mechanism at play that is of relevance to us is the repeated shaking of a small child when grabbed around its torso leading to rib/spine/neck injuries, coup-contrecoup brain injury, and acceleration-deceleration forces within the vitreoretinal interface. There are a few other theories on why retinal haemorrhages occur, but currently this is the most widely accepted theory.

The prevalence of retinal haemorrhages is highest in children under 3 years of age and is not commonly reported in older children. The incidence of intracranial injury secondary to abusive head trauma is highest in infancy (<12 months old). It is harder to inflict a shaking injury on older, heavier children with stronger neck muscles, especially as they also have a smaller head to body size ratio when compared to infants.

If the paediatric team has started the process, there will be safeguarding barriers put in place. This may vary between Trusts but usually implies that a health care or social worker escorts the child to the outpatient visit or stays bedside with the patient 24/7 whilst the parents are present. The preliminary safety assessment performed by the safeguarding team decides on the level of precautions required. In cases where the child or other children are felt to be in an immediate position of risk, child protection services move in within the day to move them to a position of safety until the situation has been de-escalated or the diagnosis excluded. If there is strong preliminary evidence of foul play, it is not uncommon to have to examine the child with police officer observers.

What certainly does not happen is a child turning up to the outpatients from home or returning straight home after the eye clinic visit! A child cannot be discharged to the community until the NAI diagnosis is ruled out.

The entire process is usually emotionally challenging, not just for the family involved but sometimes for the professionals who become involved in the child's care. There is an inherent instinct to protect society's young, especially amongst healthcare professionals, and the thought of a helpless child being physically shaken up so much that their retinas bleed and their brains swell up can affect even the most hardened among us. These complex feelings are often foreign territory for an ophthalmologist.

Non-accidental injury or abusive head trauma are sensitive terms so care should be taken not to flaunt these terms in a busy waiting room or leave derivatives of the word 'abuse' in parts of notes with easy access to uninvolved personnel, such a post-it note on front of notes for example. The process should be transparent. The family is aware of why the child is having these investigations, but it is worth reiterating that the purpose of your examination is to rule out eye signs that could be present as part of the child's present condition.

Regardless of the background story, one should treat the situation objectively. Remember that our priority is to obtain a high quality examination of the patient in a process which minimises stress or harm.

In the rare situation where you, the ophthalmologist, are the first professional to suspect a safeguarding issue after a child presents to eye casualty brought directly by the parents, the first person to inform is your consultant for advice followed by the local Trusts' named safeguarding officers who could either be a nurse or a consultant (commonly a consultant paediatrician).

DIFFERENTIAL DIAGNOSIS

Birth haemorrhage, Bleeding dyscrasias (e.g. Von Williebrand disease's, protein C deficiency), Leukemia: These can mimic retinal haemorrhages in shaken baby syndrome (SBS), but birth haemorrhages tend to resolve around 2–4 weeks from birth, and leukemia and blood dyscrasias can be excluded with haematological testing.

Accidental injury and short distance falls: In rare cases, accidental falls especially those associated with subdural haematoma can have unilateral, localised and superficial retinal haemorrhages. Crush injuries however have been reported to produce haemorrhages similar to those seen in shaken baby syndrome.

Seizures: These are rarely associated, and if they do occur it may be secondary to a head injury sustained from the seizure. Retinal haemorrhages associated with convulsions are few and are close to the optic discs.

Cardiopulmonary resuscitation: Very unlikely, even if done by unskilled individuals.

Choking, gagging, and vomiting: Very rare, if they occur at all.

Apparent life threatening event (ALTE): No previous reported associations.

Vaccinations: No previous reported associations.

High cervical injuries: No evidence that high cervical injury alone can cause retinal haemorrhages.

Raised intracranial pressure: A dramatic rise in intracranial pressure may produce unilateral or bilateral retinal bleeds similar to those seen in abusive head trauma.

Conditions causing retinal haemorrhages: The following have been reported in literature but are found in small case series' or even single case reports only. Some of these will not pose a clinical dilemma as there will be other diagnostic clues in the systemic examination and most of these do not have the multiple and peripheral widespread multi-layered haemorrhages seen in abusive head trauma.

Haemorrhagic disease of the newborn, sickle cell retinopathy, ECMO treatment, retinopathy of prematurity, galactosemia, Henoch–Schönlein purpura, thrombocytopaenic purpura, maternal ingestion of cocaine, meningitis, intracranial vascular malformation, optic disc drusen, tuberous sclerosis, xlinked retinoschisis, intraocular surgery, severe hypertension, homocystinuria, glutaric aciduria, osteogenesis imperfecta, osteoporosis-pseudoglioma syndrome, incontinentia pigmenti, central retinal vein occlusion, infections, fibromuscular dysplasia, Terson's syndrome, asphyxia, RetCam screening.

CLINICAL EXAMINATION

There is trepidation when it comes to examining small infants and young children.

Referring a patient to be examined by your senior or consultant colleague is sometimes necessary in cases of very young babies or when examination is difficult. However, unless you think you are doing harm to a child, an ophthalmology trainee of any level should always attempt the examination first. It is not uncommon for apprehensive trainees to avoid examining babies during the earlier years of their training, and then end up as a senior doctor never having examined an infantile retina before.

There is no consensus on an age cut off so any child who has been flagged up with a NAI query should have an examination by the ophthalmology team (a positive finding in a child older than 2 years old would be unlikely). The examination should be done as soon as is practical, within the same day if possible, and certainly before discharge. The ophthalmology examination, however, should NOT be used as a screening tool before the paediatric team instigates NAI investigations.

In some units, there may be local policy that dictates that all NAI cases go directly to a paediatric ophthalmologist especially in highly suspicious cases.

Other ocular signs of abusive head trauma do exist such as subconjunctival haemorrhages, lid ecchymoses, lid oedema, chemosis, abrasions, orbital fractures and anterior segment injury. These findings should be looked for during the examination. The RCOPHTH proforma (see Figure 20.1) acts as an aide-memoire.

RECORDING OF OPHTHAMOLOGICAL FEATURES IN SUSPECTED PAEDIATRIC HEAD TRAUMA

HISTORY — Continue on reverse

PATIENTS DETAILS

If possible to assess

| Visual acuity | Right eye | Left eye |

OCULAR MOTILITY

Right eye   Left eye

Pupil size and Pupillary reflexes

PERIOCULAR BRUISING: (mark areas of bruising)

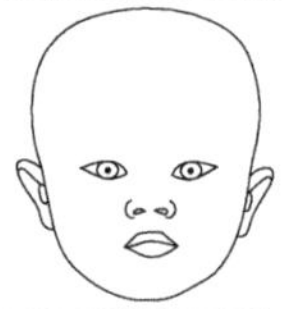

SUBCONJUNCTIVAL HAEMORRHAGES

| Right eye | | Left eye | |
| Yes | No | Yes | No |

ANTERIOR SEGMENT

| Right Eye | Left Eye |

Pupils dilated with

FUNDUS Circle if present	**RIGHT** EYE				**LEFT** EYE			
Retinal haemorrhages	YES		NO		YES		NO	
NUMBER of Retinal haemorrhage	Few (1–10)	Many (10–20)	Too numerous to count		Few (1–10)	Many (10–20)	Too numerous to count	
LOCATION of retinal haemorrhages	Pre retinal	Intraretinal	Subretinal	Multilayered	Pre retinal	Intraretinal	Subretinal	Multilayered
DISTRIBUTION of retinal haemorrhages	Posterior Pole Few/many/ too numerous to count (Zone 1-ROP classification)		Periphery Few/many/ too numerous to count (outside Zone 1)		Posterior Pole Few/many/ too numerous to count (Zone 1-ROP classification)		Periphery Few/many/ too numerous to count (outside Zone 1)	
SIZE of retinal haemorrhages	Small (< 1dd)	Medium 1–2dd	Large >2dd		Small (<1dd)	Medium 1-2dd	Large >2dd	
MORPHOLOGY of haemorrhages White centered or other								
Macula retinoschisis								
Perimacular folds								
Optic disc								
OTHER findings								

Circle single or multiple appropriate responses if present enter free text

| Name and signature | **Fundus examined with** Indirect ophthalmoscope (and 20d / 28d / 30d/ 2.2d) |
| Date and time of examination | Retcam ☐   **OR**   Photography ☐ OCT ☐ |

Figure 20.1 Royal College of Ophthalmologists NAI Proforma.

History (cont.)

Other findings

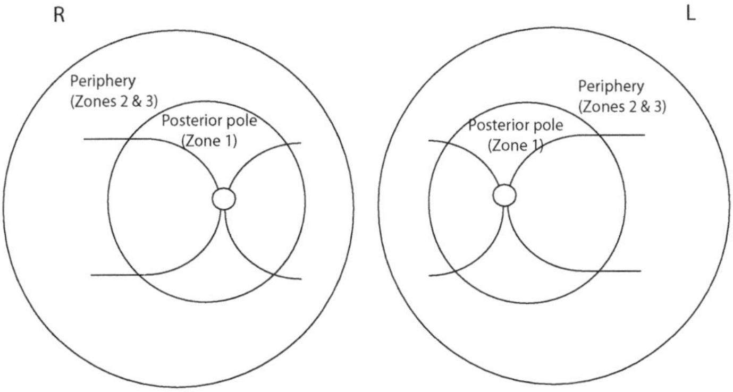

R   L

Periphery
(Zones 2 & 3)
  Posterior pole
  (Zone 1)

Periphery
(Zones 2 & 3)
  Posterior pole
  (Zone 1)

Comments

Name

Signature

Figure 20.1 (Continued)   Royal College of Ophthalmologists NAI Proforma.

Location: Occasionally, early on in the presentation, some of these children may be intubated in a paediatric intensive care unit. The astute registrar would use this opportunity to examine the baby, and the task becomes no harder than an indirect ophthalmoscopic examination on a model eye.

If the patient requires a magnetic resonance imaging (MRI) or a computed tomography (CT) scan under a general anaesthestic, this can be a good opportunity to do a dilated examination, preferably in the anaesthetic room before the scan.

Most departments would facilitate this as combined procedures done in one sitting are in the interests of the patient.

If the above situations are not feasible, and there are no clinical reasons why the child cannot be brought to an outpatient environment, then it is not unreasonable to examine the patient in the eye clinic or eye casualty setting.

Equipment and technique: If the baby is fully awake, paediatric ophthalmology experience comes in handy. Skill with the indirect ophthalmoscope is required and any condensing lens could be used as long as the view is adequate (20D/28D/30D/2.2D). Techniques include:

- Examining a baby wrapped up in a bundle in a cot (see Figure 20.2a).

- Examining a baby with the knees to knees technique (see Figure 20.2b).

- Examining a toddler sitting up on a parent's lap ± mild restraining of the head and arms (see Figure 20.2c).

- For most infants under 12 weeks old, anaesthetic drops (oxybuprocaine 0.4% or proxymetcaine 0.5%) and a neonatal speculum could be utilised if done with care. One should always attempt examining without a speculum first in all cases.

- In older infants once they reach a certain strength and size, a speculum may cause considerable stress, and thus the 'finger speculum' may be more appropriate (Figure 20.3a and b).

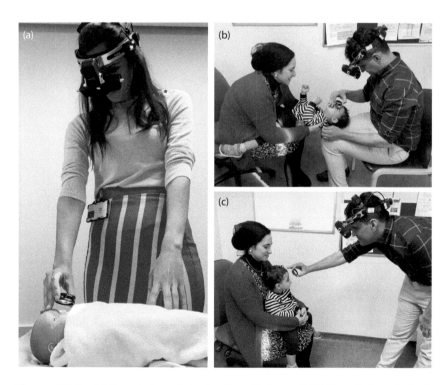

Figure 20.2 (a) Examining a baby in a bundle in a cot. (b) Examining a baby in a knees to knees position. (c) Examining a toddler in a parent's embrace.

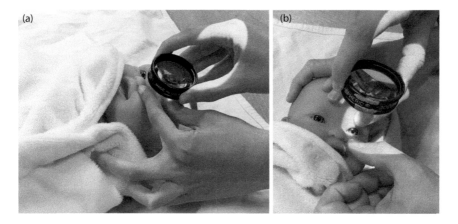

Figure 20.3 (a) Examiner using two fingers to hold apart eyelids; (b) assistant using two thumbs to hold apart eyelids.

- Scleral indentation to view peripheral retina (like in retinopathy of prematurity screening) is NOT necessary in NAI examinations as the lesions will never be in the far periphery alone.

- In older children who can sit on a table mounted slit lamp, formal examination is more typical. These are the children who are not likely to have any retinal haemorrhages due to their age and a good quality examination to confirm this should be achievable.

Imaging options: Increasingly, it is becoming important to image the retina especially in eyes with positive findings. It is one of the most crucial pieces of evidence in cases which end up in court. Modalities include:

1. Contact widefield (e.g. PanoCam, ICON, NEOcam, RetCam [Figure 20.4]).
2. Scanning laser ophthalmoscopy (SLO) ultra widefield camera (Optos, Optos Inc, Dunfermline).
3. Slit lamp mounted fundus camera (e.g. TOPCON, Zeiss).
4. Portable optical coherence tomography (OCT) (Bioptigen, Inc).

The limitation here is the availability of these machines as they are costly and not all units would have one. A large proportion of positive findings would be found in children who are sedated or intubated, and in these situations a contact widefield camera like the RetCam (Figure 20.4) is ideal. It could be performed in awake babies with anaesthetic drops, a speculum, and an assistant to hold the child's head and body. A minimum of five photographs should be obtained (posterior pole, superior, temporal, inferior, nasal). Some experience with the contact-type camera is recommended as prolonged examinations can cause stress to the child.

In awake patients, children as young as 2 can be coaxed into having their retinas photographed on a quick acquisition SLO camera like the Optos. This requires some experience from the ophthalmic technician.

In cases with no findings, if it is practical to do so (e.g. a cooperative 4-year-old), it is worth taking a baseline retinal photo as evidence to confirm your examination. OCT is a useful tool to evaluate the vitreoretinal interface, but currently most units do not have a handheld OCT.

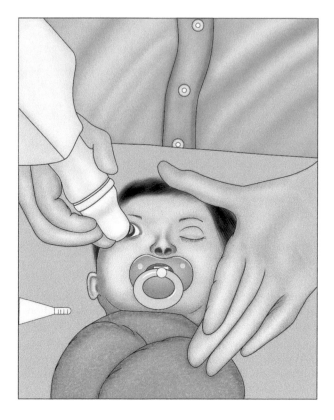

Figure 20.4   An ophthalmologist using a RetCam handpiece.

Good quality imaging does not replace good documentation however. Every entry needs to be dated, signed and legible, which is important when either yourself or a colleague has to review the notes retrospectively and generate a report.

DIAGNOSIS

There are still controversies around retinal haemorrhages in abusive head trauma, a lot of which are beyond the scope of this chapter. There is no defining feature, and retinal haemorrhages can occur in other forms of trauma, accidental or otherwise. The diagnosis is based on a multi-disciplinary approach taking into account the history and the absence/presence of the other stigmata of NAI.

There are no ocular findings that are pathognomonic for abusive head trauma but multi-layered bilateral, retinal haemorrhages involving the posterior pole and the periphery are highly suggestive of it.

MANAGEMENT

The ophthalmologists' key role is diagnosis and detailed clinical documentation. This role however cannot be underestimated as NAI is a very complex condition. Every process of the pathway needs to be carried out speedily in order for local authorities to make decisions about the necessity and speed in which to escalate child protection services. Delay in one cog of the wheel can in turn cause systemic delays that take up to days. As mentioned previously, this is not ideal when a child or other young children's safety may be at stake.

Conversely in situations where the NAI protocol has been initiated by the paediatric team in an otherwise well child, a delay in a retinal examination could lead to a prolonged period of stress for a family with the child likely kept in an acute hospital bed unnecessarily.

There is no treatment specific for retinal haemorrhages during the acute phase. However, children who survive need to be monitored for visual development issues such as amblyopia, strabismus and cerebral visual impairment, especially if concomitant brain injury was present.

In cases of non-resolving visually obscuring preretinal or vitreous haemorrhage, macula hole, or retinal detachment, there could be a role for vitreoretinal surgery. However, paediatric vitrectomies especially in infants are fraught with risks, and it would be uncommon to find a case with a convincing benefit: risk ratio.

FOLLOW UP

Retinal haemorrhages will disappear with time (2–4 weeks). A follow-up examination can give vital functional and structural information. Electrodiagnostic testing is indicated if there is evidence of impaired vision.

If there were no retinal haemorrhages seen and no significant positive findings in the brain, the child may be discharged.

PITFALLS

1. Inadequate documentation.
2. Not taking the opportunity to examine the child when they are still intubated.
3. Not imaging the retina even if the resources are available.

FURTHER READING

Adams G. et al. Update from the ophthalmology child abuse working party: Royal College of Ophthalmologists. *Eye (Lond)*. 2004;18(8):795–798.

The Ophthalmology Child Abuse Working Party, Childabuse and the eye. *Eye*. 1999;13:3–10.

The Royal College of Ophthalmologists Clinical Guidance, Abusive head trauma and the eye in infancy. 2013. https://www.rcophth.ac.uk/wp-content/uploads/2014/12/2013-SCI-292-ABUSIVE-HEAD-TRAUMA-AND-THE-EYE-FINAL-at-June-2013.pdf

21 One or Both Optic Discs are Swollen

Tariq Mohammad

KEY POINTS

1. Ensure baseline fundus photographs/OCT disc are taken on first presentation if available
2. Do not confuse a crowded disc, optic disc drusen and tilted discs with true optic disc swelling
3. Positive spontaneous venous pulsation does not completely rule out true disc swelling
4. GCA is a clinical diagnosis and a normal ESR and/or CRP doesn't rule out GCA

DIAGRAM OF ALGORITHM

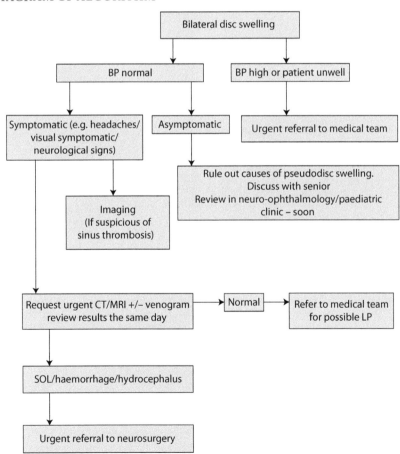

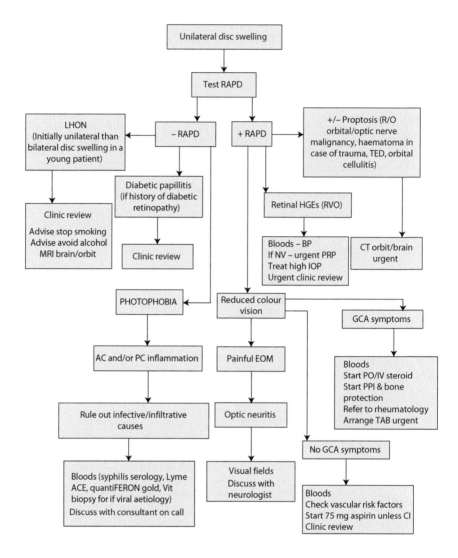

REFERRAL AND PRESENTATION

Papilloedema (PE) implies bilateral disc swelling secondary to raised intracranial pressure (ICP), whereas optic disc swelling refers to optic disc oedema secondary to other causes. These terminologies are, however, not well recognised and therefore the title of most referrals will be papilloedema which could mean unilateral or bilateral disc swelling, or indeed any form of disc swelling whatsoever.

Patients can present with a wide range of symptoms of varying severity and therefore a detailed history including drug use as well as dietary habits is paramount to help reach a sensible working diagnosis.

Headaches (see Chapter 22): Optic disc swelling associated with headaches may indicate a sinister pathology with raised ICP caused by a space occupying lesion (SOL) or intracranial bleed. Specific headache history should be taken to identify worrying features such as a severe thunderclap or a new onset early morning headache, one that wakes the patient from sleep for example. A temporal ache in a young or elderly patient will most likely be referred as giant cell arteritis (GCA), and the patient may have already started on oral steroids. This doesn't necessarily mean they have GCA; therefore, a through ocular examination with an open mind is warranted. GCA is exceedingly rare in patients <50 years of age and in certain ethnicities.

Visual symptoms: In the acute phase, visual acuity may not be affected in PE, however in cases of disc swelling secondary to other causes, there may be a change in visual acuity. Approximately 70% of patients with idiopathic intracranial hypertension (IIH) may describe a transient visual obscuration that usually occurs with changes in posture and may be unilateral or bilateral. Blind spot enlargement may be the only visual field defect in the acute phase depending on the severity of disc swelling. However, in severe cases peripheral visual field constriction or arcuate scotoma involving the inferior nasal field may occur worryingly due to infarction or ischaemia of the optic nerve.

Diplopia: Motility deficits may be seen as a false localising sign in patients with raised ICP due to involvement of unilateral and/or bilateral abducens (sixth) nerve palsy. This is due to stretching of sixth cranial nerve over the petrous part of the temporal bone. The incidence of a sixth cranial nerve palsy in patients with IIH is around 38%. Patients usually report a horizontal diplopia. Third and fourth cranial nerve palsies, although not common, can also be present in IIH.

DIFFERENTIAL DIAGNOSIS

It is important to differentiate between true papilloedema (PE) and pseudo-papilloedema as misdiagnosis can lead to unnecessary imaging and invasive procedures in the latter. The key is the presence or absence of raised ICP, of which there are many causes, including idiopathic intracranial hypertension (IIH), venous sinus thrombosis, a tumour or other space occupying lesion and so forth.

The exact list is not essential to know as your job in eye casualty is to recognise this and pass the patient on to the appropriate team. Pseudo-PE aetiology can range from; diabetes, Leber's hereditary optic neuropathy (LHON) to retinal vein occlusion but again, your task is to differentiate PE from pseudo causes and pass the patient on, not to investigate everything possible.

Optic disc drusen (ODD): Common cause of asymptomatic optic disc 'swelling' or pseudo-PE in children is with an incidence of 0.34%–2.4%. ODD in children are buried and calcified, which makes the initial diagnosis on the slit lamp challenging. Moreover, PE and ODD may coexist in which case other clinical signs and symptoms must be considered.

Congenital full disc (CFD): Another common presentation is a 'crowded disc' or a CFD. A CFD is where normal number of axons exit through a small scleral canal giving a false appearance of a swollen disc, commonly associated with hypermetropia.

Tilted discs: Either a vertical or oblique axis is not so common, but certainly gives the appearance of a swollen disc due to sectoral elevation that may be confused with early disc swelling, common in myopes.

Unilateral or bilateral disc swelling can be present due to a wide range of ocular and systemic conditions. Generally, these can be classified into ischaemic, vascular, inflammatory, infective, infiltrative and compressive aetiology (VITAMIN).

Ischaemia: Arteritic (GCA) or non-arteritic causes (ischaemic optic neuropathy [NAION]) of optic nerve inflammation exist. GCA is the one of the very few ophthalmic emergencies that must be ruled out in an elderly patient with unilateral disc swelling with associated systemic features. NAION is associated with a history of vascular risk factors, absence of GCA symptoms and the presence of an altitudinal field defect. It is not reliably possible to tell the difference between the two causes by simply looking at the nature of the swollen disc.

Vascular: Unilateral optic disc swelling associated with retinal haemorrhages in one or more quadrants or vascular tortuosity may be associated with retinal vascular disease. An impending CRVO or CRVO may have signs of obscured optic disc margins with haemorrhage giving the appearance of pseudo-PE. Prolonged, untreated, raised ICP however may as a consequence cause a CRVO, so don't ignore the symptoms of a headache. Watch out for malignant hypertension and diabetes as causes as well, so measure BP and BM, though it would be unusual for these conditions to only affect one eye.

Inflammation: May involve the anterior and/or posterior segment. Demyelination is the most common cause of optic nerve inflammation (optic neuritis). Typically a young patient will present with a dramatic loss or reduction in vision with pain on eye movements. The optic neuritis treatment trial (ONTT) showed that the use of oral steroids only speeds up the visual recovery and doesn't affect the final visual outcome. This should be discussed with the patient and a prompt referral to an on call neurologist is warranted. These patients mostly undergo an MRI of the brain to rule out demyelinating processes as well as to determine the future risks of multiple sclerosis. The risk of MS at 15 years increases from 25% to 72%, if there are more than one white matter lesion on the MRI brain scan.

Patients with an infective aetiology in addition to reduced VA may also present with photophobia due to inflammatory cells in the aqueous or vitreous humour. These patients should undergo urgent blood testing to find the infective organism and immune status before commencing any potential treatment. These patients should be discussed with a senior or consultant. Infiltrative conditions include sarcoidosis and leukaemia. Compressive lesions are not common causes of optic disc swelling but must be discussed with the supervising consultant. Your role is not to find the exact cause but to diagnose or rule out papilloedema and to pass the rest in an appropriate direction.

CLINICAL EXAMINATION
Don't forget general examination and recording vital signs so as not to miss raised blood pressure as a cause of pseudo-PE. Clinical ocular examination includes functional (VA, colour vision, pupil assessment, VF) and structural assessment of the optic nerve.

Functional Assessment of the Optic Nerve
Visual acuity (VA): VA is usually recorded by the nurses before patient is seen in clinic; however, repeat VA yourself if your clinical findings don't match the VA you expect for that patient. VA may or may not be affected, depending on cause and severity.

Pupils: Absolute (AAPD) and relative afferent pupillary defects (RAPD): AAPD means complete loss of optic nerve function, whereas RAPD means partial loss of optic nerve function in relation to the fellow eye. Therefore RAPD is commonly seen in unilateral optic neuropathy and will not be present in symmetrical, bilateral conditions. It may also be present in unilateral retinal disease, however, the retinal pathology has to be quite severe to have a clinically evident RAPD. In AAPD the pupil size is symmetrical with no response to bright light in either eye when the affected pupil is stimulated. When bright light is shown to unaffected eye there is constriction in both eyes as well as intact normal near reflex. RAPD testing relies on a normal contralateral eye and direct and consensual reflex are normal in both eyes. RAPD can be elicited by performing swinging test where both pupils dilate when bright light is shown to the affected eye. Always check for an APD/RAPD yourself, when you suspect optic nerve pathology.

Dyschromatopsia: Red and green colour deficiency is usually acquired and can be a sign of optic nerve dysfunction. It can be tested using Ishihara pseudo-isochromatic test plates. Plate one (number 12) of the Ishihara test should be read by all patients whether they are partial or completely colour blind. Red desaturation can be assessed through monocular comparison of a red hat pin or equivalent object.

Visual field (VF): Confrontational VF is more reliable for gross defects such as a hemianopias and less so for subtle arcuate defects. Blind spot size can be compared to your own for enlargement. Where possible, assess VF using formal Humphrey or Goldmann machines and interpret according to reliability (see Investigations).

Structural Assessment of the Optic Nerve

Optic disc measurement: This is very important in ruling out a crowded disc or CFD, with smaller, crowded discs termed a 'disc at risk' and are more vulnerable to damage. The VDD can be measured using a narrow-slit beam with either a Volk 78D lens (correction factor 1.1) or Volk 90D (correction factor 1.3) or by OCT.

Optic disc margins and blood vessels: Typically, obscuration of optic disc margins is the earliest sign and may involve one or more quadrants of the disc followed by obscuration of major blood vessels (see Figure 21.1). ODD, if visible, will appear as spherical nodules on the disc surface. Paton's lines are circumferential lines in the nearby retina seen with pressure from a nearby swollen disc.

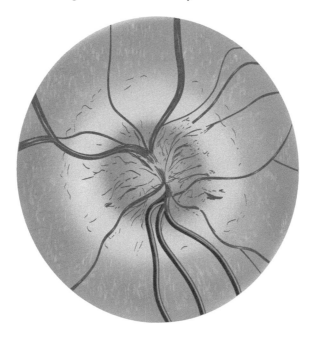

Figure 21.1 A clinically swollen optic disc.

Disc colour: Disc hyperaemia results from capillary dilatation and engorgement of its blood vessels. Retinal nerve fibre layer (RNFL) haemorrhages can be seen on the disc itself or margins (Figure 1.1). Flame shaped haemorrhages and cotton wool spots are a sign of RNFL ischaemia. CFDs also appear hyperaemic with either very small or no cup.

Spontaneous venous pulsation (SVP): This is observed as pulsatile flow within a vein on the optic nerve head. The absence of SVP is usually associated with true disc swelling, but be aware as it is also absent in 20% of the normal population.

Cranial nerve examination: Relevant cranial nerve examination must be performed that may be a consequence of the condition and help localise pathology (or not in the case of a false localising sixth CN palsy).

Perform dilated examination for other less common ocular findings associated with pseudo-PE including: macular star, choroidal folds and vitreous or retinal haemorrhages.

INVESTIGATIONS

The below investigations are helpful to differentiate between true and pseudo causes of papilloedema.

Visual fields: Where available perimetry should be performed but be aware of the high fixation losses (>20%) and high false positives (>15%) indices as this would affect the reliability of the test. Goldmann or Humphrey VF 120 or 10-2 programmes are useful in demarcating and monitoring changes due to neurological causes of field loss.

B-scan ultrasound: Drusen appear as hyperechoic areas on the optic nerve head that are best identified using a low gain. In true disc swelling a crescent sign can be seen which appears as circle of fluid within the optic nerve at a standard gain. This should be performed as baseline in all uncertain cases.

Disc OCT: OCT measures nerve fibre layer thickness (NFL), optic disc size and documents a colour photograph of the optic disc for monitoring and medicolegal purposes (see Figure 21.2). Generally, the RNFL is thickened in true disc swelling whereas it is thinned in ODD. Quadrants of RNFL loss (atrophy) will also be shown.

Autofluorescence and fluorescein angiography: These methods show early optic disc leakage and early and late nodular staining in ODD. Angiography is an invasive but useful investigation in detecting PE but it may not be readily available as first line via eye casualty. OCT-A may be an alternative.

Bloods: Routine FBC for haematological conditions and for infective aetiology include syphilis, tuberculosis, Lyme disease and so forth. If you suspect optic neuritis, there are specific antibodies which should only be requested after discussion with a neurologist and senior doctor ESR and CRP are needed if an inflammatory condition is suspected.

Imaging: To exclude space occupying lesions, bleeds and hydrocephalus in symptomatic patients. Ensure there is an up-to-date eGFR in case contrast is required, which is mostly the case in these patients. Get to know your local neuroradiologist, order and chase your own cases or handover appropriately where you can't. Always look at the scans yourself as sometimes things can be missed. Refer onward depending on what is found, follow up cases with reduced optic nerve function or cranial nerve palsy.

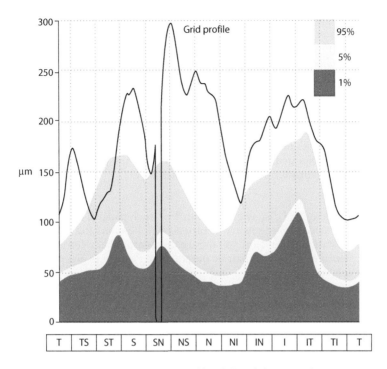

Figure 21.2 A thickness map obtained by OCT of the optic disc.

DIAGNOSIS

The main dilemma in these patients is establishing if there is a true disc swelling. Once this decision is made, working through a differential diagnosis and coming to a reasonable conclusion may not be the most difficult thing to do. The difficulty arises in cases where neither the optometrist referring clinician nor the eye casualty doctor is sure whether this is a true disc swelling or not. Such cases can take a lot longer and require a lot more investigation as wrong interpretation may either miss a sinister pathology or subject a patient to radiation and a LP when not required. Judge the urgency case by case. If there is reduction of optic nerve function, neurological signs or symptoms, or symptoms of raised intracranial pressure, perform investigations or refer urgently. The well, with minimal systemic or ocular signs or symptoms there is time, request an MRI or refer to clinic. Moreover, in cases where the patient had PE in the past, recurrent rises in ICP may not manifest as PE in the future when there has been loss of the nerves from previous damage.

OCT imaging of the discs can be handy but must not be used alone to make a diagnosis; stereoscopic examination is necessary to appreciate a raised disc. Involve a senior colleague early in such cases to avoid any delay in management.

MANAGEMENT

Papilloedema: Where non-ophthalmic pathology is suspected or found, urgent medical/neurological or neurosurgical referral is sought. The very essence of your role in dealing with this sign is to find true PE and treat it as the emergency that it is.

Pseudo-PE: Management is utterly dependent on the specific cause. GCA should be managed in conjunction with your rheumatology or medical team depending on local protocols, according to which prompt steroid treatment should be commenced. Potential treatment options include high dose oral steroids or IV methyprednisolone with bone and GI protection. Senior review should be sorted for urgent TAB and steroid management (again dependent on local protocols). Malignant hypertension requires immediate referral to medical teams.

For all borderline asymptomatic cases, it may be reasonable to monitor these patients with serial OCT disc, though never in eye casualty. If in doubt, speak to a senior. Patients with normal optic nerve function, no neurological symptoms and ODD can be discharged, with information given to the patient so they don't get referred back again after their next sight test.

FOLLOW UP

Where the aetiology of disc swelling is unclear, such patients should be seen by a consultant or senior colleague in an outpatient clinic soon after initial discussion at first presentation. The majority of these patients are either referred to paediatric, medical, neuro team or ophthalmic outpatients. Priority is given to those with optic nerve compromise.

PITFALLS

1. The main pitfall is obviously missing a true disc swelling, which can be associated with sight and life threatening complications.
2. Most young patients undergo unnecessary imaging for an undiagnosed drusen which is traumatic for the patient and parents. Avoid this by simply taking an extra step and performing: B-scan/OCT/AF or OCT-A.
3. A small proportion of patients will have normal ESR and/or CRP; therefore, treat GCA if there is high clinical suspicion and arrange an urgent TAB.

FURTHER READING

Wills Eye Institute, 2016. *The Wills Eye Manual: Office and Emergency Room Diagnosis and Treatment of Eye Disease*, Wolters Kluwer.

22 Headaches and Pain in the Temple

Bhavna Kumari Sharma

KEY POINTS

1. Urgent ESR or plasma viscosity, CRP and FBC are essential for a when giant cell arteritis (GCA) is considered a viable diagnosis – always chase the result before leaving work as GCA is a systemic, fatal illness if left untreated. Early recognition is crucial to prevent irreversible ischaemia and loss of vision to one or both eyes.
2. Be aware! GCA can still present in patients younger than 50 years with normal ESR, CRP and biochemistry values so treat the patient and not the 'numbers'. Counsel your patients appropriately.
3. Any sudden-onset, acute, 'thunderclap' or 'worst headache of my life', especially with ptosis or ophthalmoplegia, requires immediate triage towards an emergency department for urgent neuro-imaging.
4. You will often be the first person the patient has seen regarding their headache, so take a deep breath and a succinct history to guide your diagnosis.

DIAGRAM OF ALGORITHM

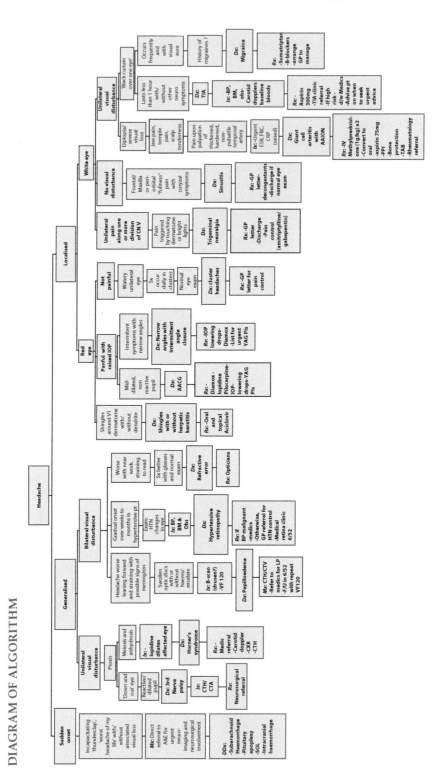

REFERRAL AND PRESENTATION

When a patient with a new onset headache is referred for urgent ocular assessment, signs of raised intracranial pressure (papilloedema, sixth CN palsy and visual field defect) or GCA is what they want to exclude. Patients with suspected GCA without ocular symptoms do not require ophthalmic evaluation. A typical referral from a GP or optician: patient over age of 50 with the following presentation (see Table 22.1).

A consultation with a patient with suspected GCA, however, may go like this:

Ethel (patient): 'I've had a headache around my right eye and this sore head for the past week.'

You: 'Oh no, that doesn't sound good. Has your vision changed with this headache, Ethel?'

Ethel: 'I was seeing sort of double of everything doc but only for the first 2 days – but now I can just see your fingers waggling from this right eye. It is all hazy. I think it is my cataracts are playing up.'

You: 'Does your jaw hurt when you chew food or talk for long periods?'

Ethel: 'Gosh, yes Doctor. Although, I haven't had much appetite with this awful headache. My shoulders are aching too.'

You: 'Does your scalp feel sore when you brush your hair?'

Ethel: 'Well I don't have much hair to brush these days but, yes, it is sore to touch on this right side now you mention it. Paracetamol has not helped. What is it Doctor?'

DIFFERENTIAL DIAGNOSIS

- Non-arteritic ischaemic optic neuropathy (NAION) – altitudinal field defect

  - Disc at risk (check size of optic disc in the fellow eye), vascular medical history (Hypertension, diabetes, high cholesterol)

  - No systemic symptoms when compared to a patient with GCA

  - Visual loss not as severe as AION/GCA

Table 22.1: Outline of the Systemic and Ocular Manifestations of Giant Cell Arteritis

Systemic Manifestations of GCA Usually Start Before Ocular Symptoms	Ocular Manifestations of GCA
<ul><li>Acute or gradual onset</li><li>New headache – temporal or occipital regions</li><li>Tenderness over the temporal artery</li><li>Scalp pain and tenderness – localised or generalised</li><li>Jaw claudication (ischaemia of masseter muscles)</li><li>Non-specific symptoms such as shoulder girdle pain, weight loss, fever, malaise and even depression</li><li>Polymyalgia rheumatica symptoms (or known PMR diagnosis)</li></ul>	<ul><li>Amaurosis fugax – transient visual loss about a week before permanent visual loss</li><li>Permanent, severe loss of vision (CF/PL/NPL) – due to optic nerve ischaemia, rarely CRAO</li><li>Second eye involvement commonly occurs within 2 weeks</li><li>Other associated ocular symptoms include: Diplopia (CN palsy), eye pain, ptosis</li></ul>

- Segmental disc swelling (with or without flame haemorrhages)
- Normal ESR/CRP
- Vasculitis – RA, SLE, PAN etc
- TIA (amarousis fugax may precede optic nerve head infarction)
- Central retinal artery occlusion – usually painless loss of vision with no jaw claudication
- Ocular ischaemic syndrome
- Myasthenia gravis – diplopia and jaw claudication that shows signs of fatiguability with bilateral ptosis

CLINICAL EXAMINATION

- Examination here is targeted at ruling out GCA or sinister intracranial pathology
- General observation – is this a sick patient? Is there history of trauma? Stroke?
- Any neurological features with walking/co-ordination/limb weakness
- Look and palpate the temples for the superficial temporal artery and pulse (see Figure 22.1).
- Absent pulsation (in late cases) in a thickened, tender, inflamed and nodular superficial temporal artery (best felt directly in front of pinna)
- They usually cannot be flattened against the skull if thickened
- Visual acuity, colour vision, RAPD, IOP
- Visual fields – formal or to confrontation
- Eye movements

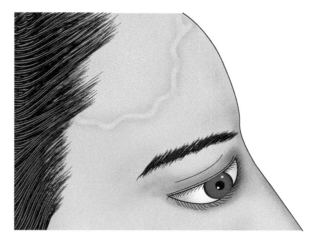

Figure 22.1 The appearance of a dilated, tortuose temporal blood vessel in a patient with giant cell arteritis.

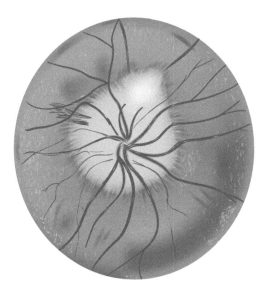

Figure 22.2 The optic disc of a patient with an anterior ischaemic optic neuropathy.

Dilated fundoscopy for signs of:

Optic nerve: Examine both eyes, observe for disc swelling, haemorrhage or pallor (see Figure 22.2). Measure the size of the unaffected disc, is it small?

Retina: Perform dilated examination after checking for a RAPD, for haemorrhages, cotton wool spots, Terson's retinopathy or vasculitis for example.

INVESTIGATIONS

Investigations and findings supporting a diagnosis of GCA include:

- Bloods:
  - ESR* or plasma viscosity: high levels of >50–60 (but can be normal in 20%–30%), CRP*: raised, FBC*: raised platelets*

- OCT optic discs and macula

- Temporal artery ultrasound – looking for vessel wall oedema/halo sign

- Temporal artery biopsy (TAB): Do not delay starting high dose steroids for a TAB. A 1-2 mm artery biopsy of the affected side should ideally be taken within 2 weeks of diagnosis. The pathologist will look for signs of granilomatous inflammation (giant cells) which may present as skip lesions.

- Intracranial Imaging: CT/MRI should be requested or via medical teams to rule out causes of headaches due to raised ICP, a SOL or inflammation.

---

* In the absence of other known systemic infections/inflammation/malignancy

Table 22.2: **The American College of Rheumatology 1990 GCA Classification Criteria**

Domain		Points	Cautions
Domain 1	1 point	New onset localized headache	No other aetiologies can better explain any one of the criteria
	1 point	Sudden onset of visual disturbances	
	2 points	Polymyalgia rheumatica (PMR)	
	1 point	Jaw claudication	Enlarged and/or pulseless temporal artery, 1 point, and tender temporal artery another 1 point
	2 points	Abnormal temporal artery	
Domain 2	1 point	Unexplained fever and/or anaemia	It must be ignored in the presence of PMR
	1 point	ESR $\geq$50 mm/hour	Vascular and/or perivascular fibrinoid necrosis along with leucocyte infiltration and granuloma
	2 points	Compatible pathology	

Note: This has a sensitivity of 93.5% and a specificity of 91.2% in diagnosing GCA, In the presence of 3 points or more out of 11 with at least one point belonging to domain 1 along with all entry criteria, the diagnosis of giant cell arteritis can be established. Entry criteria include age of greater than 50 years old without any of the exclusion criteria. Exclusion criteria consist of other ENT and eye inflammations, kidney, skin and peripheral nervous system involvement, lung infiltration, lymphadenopathies, stiff neck and digital gangrene or ulceration.

DIAGNOSIS

The diagnosis of GCA is made using a combination of clinical assessment and investigation findings. Table 22.2 indicates the diagnostic criteria according to the American Society of Rheumatologists. A positive TAB will aid diagnosis but a negative TAB does not exclude GCA.

Headaches with ocular signs associated with intracranial pathology (e.g. third or sixth CN palsy, Horner's, papilloedema) should be referred to medical teams for further investigation and urgent management.

MANAGEMENT

Early treatment of GCA is essential to prevent blindness in the fellow eye and systemic morbidity and mortality. Table 22.3 outlines the management of GCA with and without visual symptoms. Explain to your patient there is a poor prognosis for the vision in the affected eye, and intensive treatment is required to prevent loss of vision to the fellow eye.

FOLLOW UP

- Close review whilst on IV methylprednisolone to observe fellow eye

- Request urgent rheumatology review whilst inpatient or within first week of diagnosis

- Review in general or neuro-ophthalmology clinic within a month

- Advise the patient to come back urgently if they develop visual symptoms in their 'good eye'

Table 22.3: **The Management of Giant Cell Arteritis with and without Visual Symptoms**

Uncomplicated GCA (If No Visual Symptoms)	Complicated GCA (If Visual Symptoms)
1. Refer to medical team 2. Start oral prednisolone 0.75 g/kg for 4 weeks (usually 40–60 mg) 3. Reduce down by 10 mg every 2 weeks up to 20 mg 4. Reduce by 2.5 mg every 4 weeks up to 10 mg 5. Then reduce by 1 mg every 4–8 weeks depending on symptoms (relapse or not)	1. Refer to medical team 2. Admit patient for 3 pulses of IV methylprednisolone (500 mg–1 g/kg) over 3 days with cardiac monitoring 3. Then convert to oral prednislone (1 g/kg) for 4 weeks 4. Follow tapering regime as above

Adjunctive systemic medication:

1. Omeprazole 20 mg OD
   a. Start proton pump inhibitor (if patient not already on):
2. Alendronic acid 70 mg/week PO (if eGFR above 35) or Adcal D3 (colecalciferol with calcium carbonate) BD
   a. Ensure adequate bone protection:
3. Aspirin 75 mg OD

- *Remember! Rheumatology referral is essential for all patients.* These wonderful colleagues will confirm the diagnosis, taper the steroids and review the patient systemically
  - Ensure referral is sent when you see the patient – whether this be in clinic or OOH – it is something easily missed but essential and makes your life easier when it comes to systemic management of patients

Temporal artery biopsy (TAB): Who performs this is depends on your hospital pathway

1. Should always be considered in suspected GCA cases (particularly if ESR and CRP normal)
2. *However, this should not delay the prompt institution of high-dose steroid therapy*
3. Warn patient that it is diagnostic, NOT therapeutic
4. Should be performed within first 2 weeks of diagnosis
5. Biopsy specimens should be no less than 1 cm, ideally greater than 2 cm, in length
6. Contra-lateral biopsy is usually not required
7. Patients with negative TAB but a typical clinical picture and response to steroids should be regarded as having GCA

LITTLE, BUT IMPORTANT, ADVICE

- Just a note on counselling of little Ethel: often these patients do not initially comprehend that once their vision has been affected, it will not recover, and the steroid regime is to protect their fellow eye and body from further inflammatory insult.

- As mentioned previously, GCA *usually* presents in the older population, and they often come to us once the damage has been done to their vision (at least in one eye) – do not underestimate how life changing this presentation, and subsequently, this diagnosis is.

- This is particularly poignant in those patients that are already monthly regulars at the macular clinic for their fellow eye or have other such pre-existing visual impairment.

- Take a succinct social history – who do they live with at home? Do they drive? Do they have any dependents? Do they walk unaided? Do they need help in these areas?

- As ophthalmologists, we do not simply observe and treat the eyes (and perhaps the bits attached in the skull); we get the nursing staff involved to help show us how to fill out an occupational health referral form!

- Take your time to counsel the patient and do not be afraid to ask for a senior review at any stage – no question is a stupid question.

PITFALLS

1. Patients can have a dense cataract obscuring view of the disc with normal (ish) blood results but present with symptoms as listed. You are probably not sure if the optic disc is swollen or not. In this case, it is important to obtain a senior review (even if it can only be over the phone, and be honest about your findings).
2. If this is a nigh on impossible task, then trust your clinical judgement (and this chapter) and err on side of caution – treat with steroids, or discuss the case with your medical/rheumatology team.
3. Follow up such patients in 24–48 hours (if not being admitted for IV methylprednislone) to ensure symptoms are resolving on treatment – if so – then it is likely GCA and proceed as above.
4. Patients with known IIH/shunts should be discussed with neurology.
5. Raised intracranial pressure can cause CRVOs.
6. However, for those tricky customers that have symptoms that do not improve, consider investigating for the potential differential diagnoses listed in the algorithm and above.

FURTHER READING

Buttgereit F., C. Dejaco, E. L. Matteson, B. Dasgupta. Polymyalgia rheumatica and giant cell arteritis: A systematic review. *JAMA*. 315(22): 2016 Jun 14; 2442–2458.

Unwin B., C. M. Williams, W. Gilliland. Polymyalgia rheumatica and giant cell arteritis. *Am Fam Physician*. 74(9): 2006 Nov 1; 1547–1554.

23 Managing Ocular Trauma

Bhavin Patel

KEY POINTS

1. Open globe injury is a sight threatening emergency
2. Ocular trauma is classified by the Birmingham Eye Trauma Terminology System (BETTS)
3. Thorough assessment is essential pre-operatively
4. Comprehensive documentation and explanation of the risks and benefits whilst consenting patients avoids medicolegal issues

DIAGRAM OF ALGORITHM

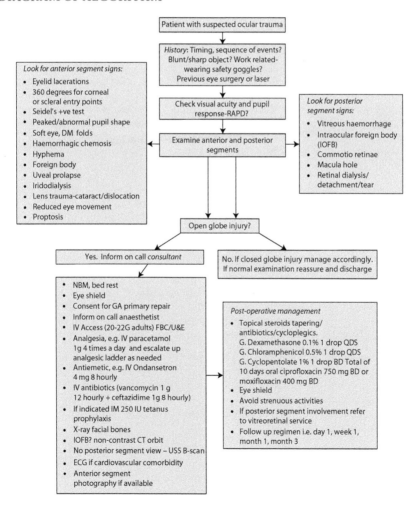

REFERRAL AND PRESENTATION

Ocular trauma potentially can be a sight threatening pathology that requires swift evaluation and management. In the context of an event causing trauma to the eye, it commonly presents as a painful, red, sometimes light sensitive, eye with deteriorating vision. The vast majority of patients present to an accident and emergency department or, depending on location, a minor injury unit where an initial assessment is attempted, often without vision being checked (or presented upside down), followed by expeditious referral to the on call registrar. A slim few patients do very little in the way of seeking medical attention as they believe their symptoms will pass and present much later to their GP or even an optician as their vision is not improving, generally with an infected or irreversibly damaged eye by that stage. Generally speaking, this happens infrequently as trauma to the eye hurts. As a rule of thumb, a painful red eye with poor vision in the context of trauma should be taken seriously and assessed accordingly.

DIFFERENTIAL DIAGNOSIS

Ocular trauma implies damage inflicted to the eyeball, soft tissues or surrounding bony structures resulting in a painful red eye with deteriorating vision. Trauma can cause a myriad of complications from a superficial abrasion, traumatic iritis or hyphaema, for example, all of which can be confirmed or excluded on slit lamp examination.

CLINICAL EXAMINATION

The first step is to measure and record visual acuity and record the presence or absence of an RAPD. If you suspect globe rupture, it is important to use minimal pressure whilst examining the eye as this could further expel intraocular contents. Slit lamp findings can be categorised into anterior and posterior segment signs. Remember to examine both eyes, documenting the time and date you started and finished your examination. Be as detailed as you can in case you are requested further down the line to produce a police report. This is not an infrequent occurrence at all.

Blunt trauma: Measure and document corneal, conjunctival tissue loss and hyphaema size. Look at how and whether the iris reacts to light and presence of transillumination defects. Traumatic mydriasis causes the iris to become frozen or poorly reactive. Dilated examination of the fundus is essential to rule out retinal pathology that would require urgent VR intervention such as RD, tear or dialysis. Document signs of Berlin's oedema or commotio retinae, choroidal rupture and large haemorrhages.

Penetration of the cornea: Penetration of the cornea through laceration or intraocular foreign body (IOFB) entry can be identified by using the Seidel test. This test is undertaken by applying fluorescein 2% to the cornea and then, with the cobalt blue filter, watching for a waterfall of aqueous fluid trickling down.

A tear drop pupil: A tear drop pupil is another sign associated with an open globe injury with the peak corresponding to the area where the iris has moved from a high pressure gradient to a low pressure gradient to seal the perforation and prevent further collapse of the eye (see Figure 23.1). This may be found in combination with a soft eye, deep AC and posterior globe rupture on CT when an IOFB or blunt trauma is suspected.

Uveal prolapse: Uveal prolapse is a sign of globe rupture where uveal tissue protrudes through an opening in the sclera. The weakest areas of the eye where the globe is likely to rupture include recti muscle insertion points, the limbus and sites of previous surgery such as corneal grafts.

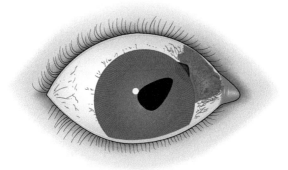

Figure 23.1 Peaked pupil after globe rupture.

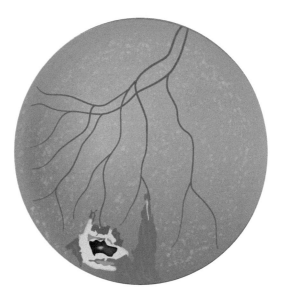

Figure 23.2 An intraocular foreign body embedded in the retina.

Intraocular foreign bodies (IOFB): Intraocular foreign bodies are commonly found in the retina although can also be found lying on the iris, in the angle or in the lens itself. If not obscured by vitreous haemorrhage, an IOFB can be viewed on slit lamp retinal examination (see Figure 23.2). Equally, if an IOFB is in the angle, perform gonioscopy if hyphaema isn't clouding the view. Perform a B-scan where an IOFB is suspected but you have a poor view of the retina.

INVESTIGATIONS

Imaging: If not performed in the A+E department, request a CT orbits, which is useful in locating an IOFB as well as other orbital injuries.

Ultrasound B-scan: Ultrasound B-scan is particularly useful where the poster segment cannot be viewed to exclude a retinal detachment or IOFB.

Other tests include basic bloods such as full blood count, urea and electrolytes, and if indicated an ECG are all important in assessing patient fitness for surgery. These are interpreted by our anaesthetic colleagues so as a proactive trainee arranging them in a timely fashion will go a long way.

You should consider documenting visible injuries via medical photography and checking all imaging yourself; you will be surprised sometimes at the things that you see that our radiology colleagues have missed.

DIAGNOSIS

Ocular trauma is not a diagnosis as such; it is broad umbrella term for describing open and closed globe injuries. These terms sub-categorise various diagnoses within them which is highlighted in Figure 23.3 and defined in Table 23.1.

MANAGEMENT

The broad principles of immediate trauma management involve medical or surgical interventions for closed or open globe injuries.

Blunt trauma: Treat traumatic uveitis and hyphaema with intense topical steroids, but initially at a lower dose in the presence of a corneal epithelial defect. Use cycloplegia for hyphaema to prevent rebleed – common at 5 days and bed rest with large bleeds. Refer all retinal pathology to VR if surgical repair is required. Manage secondary raised IOP with topical IOP lowering drops and oral diamox if severe with subsequent urgent glaucoma review.

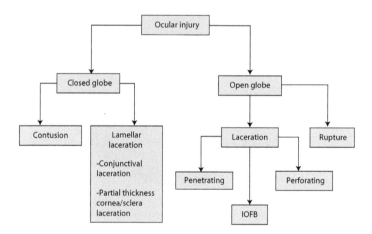

Figure 23.3 BETTS classification.

Table 23.1: **Definitions of BETTS**

Term	Definition
Open globe injury	Full thickness wound of the eye wall
Laceration	Full thickness wound caused by sharp object
Lamellar laceration	Partial thickness wound of the eye wall
Rupture	Full thickness wound of the eye wall caused by blunt trauma
Penetrating	Entrance wound present
Perforation	Entrance and exit wound present

Penetrating eye injuries: Keep the patient nil by mouth for theatre, and place a clear plastic eye shield to minimise further trauma.

- Analgesia is essential for ocular comfort, and the use of antiemetics prevent an increase in intraocular pressure and extrusion of intraocular contents from vomiting or retching.

- Antibiotics are important and it is best to start them pre-operatively, either IV or orally. Oral fluroquinolones like Ciprofloxacin 750 mg twice a day or even better Moxifloxacin 400 mg twice a day have excellent ocular penetration.

- If the wound is dirty, tetanus prophylaxis is a must which is given intramuscularly and should be strongly considered in lid lacerations.

- Post-operative topical steroids like dexamethasone 0.1% 1 drop four times a day are given on a tapering regimen for at least 4 weeks along with antibiotics like chloramphenicol 0.5% 1 drop four times a day and cycloplegics like cyclopentolate 1% 1 drop twice a day for at least 1 week.

Finally, prevention is better than cure. Education is extremely important and ensuring that protective eye wear is used in the workplace or even at home when doing particular tasks will minimise the risk of such events recurring.

FOLLOW UP

Traumatic anterior uveitis or commotio: If uncomplicated, review in 1–2 weeks in a general clinic, dilate and look at the fundus again.

Hyphaema: Review according to IOP and hyphaema size. Gonioscopy should be performed before discharging patients with blunt trauma and hyphaema.

Penetrating eye injury: Post-operative patients are generally seen at day 1 which then can extend to week 1, month 1 and month 3 should signs of improvement be seen. Intraocular pressure is also measured at each visit as topical steroids could cause this to increase.

It is important to inform the patient that if they are experiencing a painful red eye with deteriorating vision they should contact the local eye casualty so that they can be seen promptly to exclude sight threatening pathologies like endophthalmitis and sympathetic ophthalmia in the fellow eye.

PITFALLS

On the top of Mount Sinai God gave the great prophet Moses the Ten Commandments. I am neither God nor Moses, however there are *three* commandments, which if followed to the letter will steer trainees away from pitfalls.

1. **Commandment 1. Thou shall avoid making the cardinal sin**. This refers to not dilating a patient in a case of ocular trauma. It is important to identify from an early stage if there is posterior segment involvement secondary to trauma, as this requires further input from vitreoretinal specialists. Failure to do this often results in you hanging your head in shame!

2. **Commandment 2. Thou shall document to prevent**. It is important as a trainee to clearly document the patient care pathway from admission to discharge especially documenting the consent process and conversation

regarding visual prognosis. Not doing so can have medicolegal implications. To minimise this doom from occurring, have a well designed ocular trauma proforma where key information can be recorded in a useful manner, ensuring nothing is left out. Also, having anterior segment photography available enhances this documentation.

3. Lastly, **Commandment 3. Thou shall proceed with caution**. There are some circumstances where it is difficult to ascertain whether a penetrating injury has occurred. A bullous 360° subconjunctival haemorrhage in the context of trauma should be seriously considered for surgical exploration, and although CT imaging may help, nothing beats exploration under anaesthesia for definitively searching for injuries and fixing them.

FURTHER READING

Kuhn F. *Ocular Traumatology*. Springer-Verlag Berlin and Heidelberg GmbH & Co. 2008.

24 Called to ITU to Examine a Fundus

James Potts

KEY POINTS

1. Phone ahead; ITU patients may have numerous consults/procedures performed each day.
2. Examine the notes carefully; patients often have multiple pathologies giving clues about what may be found on fundal examination. The eye can be a useful diagnostic indicator in a broad spectrum of diseases.
3. Bring the relevant kit. Drops (fluorescein and dilating drops), indirect head piece, eyelid retractor and lenses. Clean all equipment before entry to ITU.
4. Perform a full anterior as well as fundal examination. ITU patients have various risk factors impairing corneal well-being which can be quickly assessed.
5. Check everything with the nurse who looks after the patient; they will know them well and highlight tubes/lines and equipment which needs avoiding.
6. Wash your hands. A lot.

DIAGRAM OF ALGORITHM

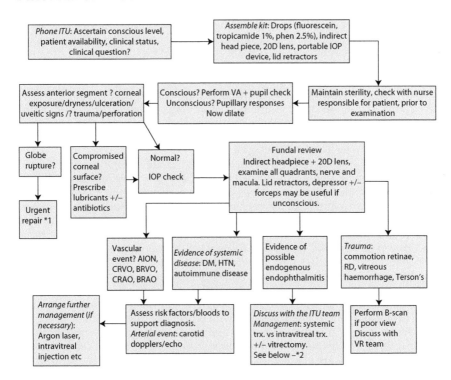

Repair of retinal detachment is, of course, an emergency and potentially sight saving, however, it will have to be weighed up against other lifesaving treatments or surgeries in the ITU patient and prioritised accordingly.

REFERRAL AND PRESENTATION

Intensive care unit (ITU) patients are the sickest in the hospital and often have numerous co-morbidities and concurrent pathologies. The eye is often not an initial priority in ITU patients. Lifesaving interventions addressing their breathing, blood pressure and kidney function come first. Intubation and sedation will also prevent ITU patients from communicating visual symptoms. Nonetheless, the eye is a highly vascularised organ and may provide useful information about previously undiagnosed systemic diseases. For the same reason, the eye is susceptible to endogenous spread from severe systemic infection.

Referral may come following the discovery of specific blood cultures, most typically candidaemia or as part of a full trauma review, especially in the context of facial trauma. If there has not been direct trauma to the globe or surrounding area, visual loss can still occur due to Purtcher's retinopathy. Purtcher's retinopathy is also found with non-traumatic cases including acute pancreatitis, renal failure, connective tissue disease and pre-eclampsia or HELLP (haemolysis, elevated liver enzymes, low platelets) syndrome, all of which are commonly seen in the ITU setting. Finally you may even be asked to review the fundus in a case of 'pyrexia of unknown origin', or 'persistent pyrexia'; candidaemia is often treated empirically in these ITU cases.

ITU patients are frequently sedated but those extubated or conscious throughout their stay may experience sudden visual loss due to vascular events. This could be secondary to blood loss, coagulopathy or emboli following surgery. Early diagnosis of central (or branch) retinal artery and vein occlusions can help limit sight loss and prevent secondary complications including rubeosis and secondary glaucoma. Not uncommonly, ITU patients may have been subjected to cranial trauma or dropped consciousness secondary to significant intracranial bleeds or stroke. This may lead to raised intracranial pressure and visual loss secondary to papilloedema or direct damage to the visual cortex within the brain. In cases of sub-arachnoid haemorrhage, between 8–18% of patients are believed to be affected by Terson's syndrome. This is a secondary vitreous haemorrhage, perhaps transmitted straight through the optic nerve head due to the dramatic change in intracranial pressure during the bleed. A thorough examination of the notes should give clues as to what may have led to the varied pathologies above.

The most common referral probably remains a fundal review following positive blood or line cultures for candidaemia or suspected candidaemia. Endogenous endophthalmitis is always a concern following candida growth on blood cultures and a fundal review is recommended by the microbiologist. However, endogenous endophthalmitis only makes up around 2%–8% of the endophthalmitis cases we see. It is always worth checking the patient hasn't had recent ophthalmic surgery or intravitreal injection to exclude exogenous endophthalmitis. Studies have suggested an increase in incidence of systemic candidaemia in recent years, likely related to an increase in the number of ITU beds, complicated surgery and prolonged ITU stays. Patients at risk of systemic candidaemia include those following major abdominal surgery, patients who have prolonged central line placement with broad spectrum antibiotic usage and to a lesser degree transplant patients and those undergoing haemofiltration/ haemodialysis. Diabetes mellitus and immunosuppression with corticosteroids and chemotherapy are also significant risk factors.

Candida is recognised as the most common cause of endogenous endophthalmitis; however, there is a gigantic range reported in the literature surrounding how frequently systemic candidaemia leads to endogenous endophthalmitis or chorioretinitis – 7%–78%. The reason for fundal review is that intraocular candidiasis is potentially blinding and may need additional treatment to the systemic anti-fungals prescribed by the ITU team. Intravitreal amphotericin or vitrectomy may be indicated with larger, sight threatening abscesses. Early ophthalmic examination may help to confirm the diagnosis in patients who are currently asymptomatic and help with prognosis and assessing treatment efficacy in those with already confirmed fungemia. It is not unusual sadly to be unable to perform definitive treatment for patients with endogenous endophthalmitis due severe systemic co-morbidity, and the general prognosis is usually but not always poor from the very beginning.

DIFFERENTIAL DIAGNOSIS

A fundal review in ITU will have a wide differential list, touched on above. When checking for signs of endogenous endophthalmitis, especially if the disease process is caught early in an asymptomatic patient, may be fairly non-specific. This would include vitreous debris or mild vitritis, cotton wool spots and subtle retinitis which could have a variety of underlying causes (see Figure 24.1). If no pre-existing systemic inflammatory disease is known, then these are often attributed to candidaemia, especially if they subsequently disappear with treatment.

Differentiating between endogenous and exogenous spread of infection is important; this usually just involves checking the patient's records for any recent ophthalmic surgical intervention combined with an anterior ophthalmic exam checking for blebs, corneal incision scars and psuedophakia (these, of course, may not be new additions).

As mentioned above, ITU patients often have multiple systemic co-morbidities; this increases the chance of finding vein and arterial occlusions as well as ischaemic

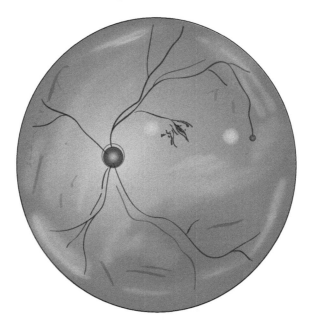

Figure 24.1 Fundoscopy in fungal endogenous endophthalmitis.

optic neuropathies. Diabetes is often a co-morbidity found with ITU patients and vitreous haemorrhage or proliferative diabetic retinopathy may be diagnosed and a differential cause of sudden visual loss.

In the context of trauma, ensuring there has not been a globe rupture, anteriorly or posteriorly, is crucial. Once this has been established, scouring the fundus for signs of retinal detachment (check for tobacco dust/blood within the vitreous), as well as any holes or tears in the peripheries is the priority. Purtscher's retinopathy is thought to be due to micro-embolism of the retinal vasculature. This can occur following long bone fractures of the lower limbs releasing fat emboli or chest and head trauma, all without direct ocular injury. Purtcher's like retinopathy can also occur following a number of significant illnesses including those detailed earlier.

A common cause of ITU admission is decreased conscious level; this may be following head injury or spontaneous intracranial bleed or ischaemic stroke. These patients are frequently intubated during admission and visual loss may only become apparent if some recovery is made and the patient extubated perhaps days or weeks later. Documenting an ophthalmic exam, which may appear normal, may be requested if these patients suffer injury to the visual cortex or optic nerves. Imaging will frequently already have been performed in these cases giving further clues.

CLINICAL EXAMINATION

Full examination in ITU will require kit to be obtained from your eye unit, including: a supply of drops (fluorescein and dilators are a must), a hand held pressure monitor to check IOP, Snellen chart and an indirect head piece with 20D lens. A trolley may be useful as dropping or losing these implements makes you very unpopular with your ward sister.

Phoning ahead will give useful tips about patient availability and their current state. Intubated/sedated patients will need lots of moving around the bed to attain adequate views, whilst aiming to avoid all tubes and lines. Sedated patients are of course extremely co-operative, making pressure taking and lid opening far less challenging. It's best to check with the patients' nurse before moving any line or touching the airway.

Start as you would in eye casualty, checking pupillary responses, their visual acuity (if awake) and performing an anterior exam with fluorescein dye. Most UK ITU settings have guidelines to try and prevent corneal exposure and secondary infection or sequelae. However, you may as well use the opportunity to check the anterior segment is normal and cornea adequately protected. If possible, an IOP check is always useful.

Next dilate the eyes to obtain adequate views, but always check if this is okay with the patient's medical team and document you have done so.

A hand held ophthalmoscope will provide reasonable information but practice with an indirect head torch and 20D lens will give wider, often more peripheral views in a shorter time period. Document your findings accurately; ophthalmic signs may be used to judge response to systemic treatment and assists your colleagues at subsequent review if you are not there.

INVESTIGATIONS AND DIAGNOSIS

Most of the ophthalmic diagnoses made in the ITU will be based on objective clinical examination.

Candida infections: Diagnosis of candidaemia is definitively made by blood culture or culture from a suspected site of involvement. Unfortunately microbiological cultures often have a relatively low yield (estimated at around 50%) and are slow to grow, often significantly lagging behind the clinical picture. With that in mind, an ocular review may be requested to support early suspicion and dilated fundal exam is recommended in all confirmed cases.

Classically, lesions from candida endophthalmitis are white/pale chorioretinal spots with fluffy or filamentous edges (see Figure 24.1). These can be isolated or multiple and associated with less specific signs including retinal haemorrhages and roth spots. More advanced disease, which is more likely to affect vision, may demonstrate severe vitritis and anterior uveitis. Macula involvement or large vitreous abscesses are also possible in these severe cases (see Figure 24.2). Embolic lesions from candidaemia have also been shown to cause conjunctivitis and episcleritis. Specific anti-fungal susceptibility testing should be requested, once a positive culture result is confirmed, as there are a variety of candida species. *Candida albicans* is the most frequent culprit (responsible for 66% of UK and 50% of US cases, according to large studies) but *C. glabrata, C. parapsilosis, C. tropicalis* and *C. krusei* are also common. *C. glabrata, C. parapsilosis* and *C. krusei* all often show resistance to azole antifungals.

If blood and line cultures are already negative or likely to have a significant delay and there is concern about candida endophthalmitis, especially in the context of vitiritis or a vitreous abscess, then a vitreous tap is advised and discussion with the vitreo-retinal team needed urgently (on the day of examination). Intubated patients in ITU with systemic and ocular candida sepsis are generally very sick with poor life expectancy.

Vascular events: Vascular events are usually fairly characteristic in their appearance and discussed in another chapter. Subtle ischaemic optic neuropathies can be challenging and need careful pupil examination and comparison with the fellow eye, optic nerve signs (pallor) may become more apparent at subsequent follow-up. Vascular occlusions, arterial or venous, all need a thorough assessment of cardiovascular risk factors; blood pressure, cholesterol, diabetes,

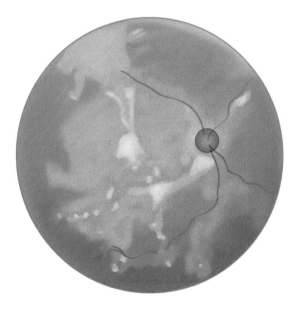

Figure 24.2   Vitreous abscess secondary to fungal endophthalmitis.

full blood count and renal function. A coagulation screen will likely already have been done in an ITU setting but worth checking. Arterial occlusions need investigation into the source of potential emboli including carotid Dopplers and echocardiogram.

Immunology: Similarly, if there is suspicion surrounding systemic auto-immune disease or poor immune response, your fundal findings may help guide further investigation. (Serum ACE/ANCA/ANA/rheumatoid factor/anti DNA/HIV – CNV/VDRL, etc.)

If there is uncertainty surrounding a potential vascular event or Purtcher's retinopathy, then OCT and FFA are helpful in differentiating between diagnoses. The reality of performing these on an acutely unwell ITU patient is unlikely; however, if the patient recovers they may be helpful for confirmation later on in an outpatient setting.

Stroke: Stroke patients or those affected by vascular events also often need formal visual fields documenting, usually following discharge from ITU. This is to help assess their ongoing needs, rehabilitation and potential ability to continue driving.

MANAGEMENT

Vitreoretinal complications: Assessment of the eye following trauma and identification of a retinal hole, tear or detachment is crucial. Liaising between the ITU team and ophthalmic VR team if a detachment is seen needs to be done immediately, especially in the context of a 'macula on' detachment. Trauma may result in posterior globe rupture as well as other presentations (see Chapter 23).

Vascular complications: Management of vascular events largely revolves around full assessment of the relevant risk factors. Early identification will help prevent a similar occurrence in the fellow eye and secondary complications.

Candida endophthalmitis: The management of candida endophthalmitis will depend on its severity as well as the clinical state of the patient. It will likely be a joint decision between the ophthalmology consultant on call, ITU team and local microbiologist. There is no single recommended treatment, but systemic anti-fungal therapy with close follow-up is advised for most cases without vitreous or macula involvement.

- In patients with milder peripheral retinal signs, systemic treatment with IV fluconazole or voriconazole is suggested. Both drugs penetrate the eye well, (especially in an inflamed eye) and can be converted to oral preparations when improvement is noted.

- Typically there is a loading dose followed by twice daily regime, (fluconazole 800 mg (12 mg/kg) loading dose, then 400–800 mg (6–12 mg/kg) once daily OR voriconazole 400 mg (6 mg/kg) IV loading dose twice daily for two doses, then 300 mg (4 mg/kg) IV or orally twice daily).

- If the patient has been recently exposed to 'azole' drugs or fluconazole resistant species is grown, then liposomal amphotericin B 3–5 mg/kg IV daily, with or without flucytosine 25 mg/kg orally 4 times daily is recommended. Amphotericin is a very toxic drug and needs monitoring.

- Patients with macular involvement and severe chorioretinitis with vitritis will need additional treatment with intravitreal amphotericin B deoxycholate 5–10 mcg/0.1 mL (sterile water) OR voriconazole 100 mcg/0.1 mL (sterile water or normal saline).

■ Those noted to have a fungal abscess or very severe disease may benefit from vitrectomy as well as intravitreal injection to decrease the organism burden within the eye.

Systemic treatment will need to continue for 4–6 weeks until resolution of all lesions is noted on repeat examination.

FOLLOW UP

Candidaemia: Fundal examination should be performed at the start of any confirmed diagnosis of candidaemia; weekly follow-up is then suggested for patients suitable for systemic treatment alone. A review of the patient on treatment completion is also advisable. Patients found to have severe vitiritis, abscesses or macula lesions requiring intravitreal treatment need much closer monitoring, likely a daily review to monitor response to treatment during the first week.

Vascular events: Patients found to have vascular events should be followed up in OPD to monitor for secondary complications, usually 4–6 weeks later. This is unless their ITU stay exceeds this and further review needs arranging on the unit. If formal visual fields are needed, ask the ITU team to phone the eye unit on discharge.

Corneal exposure: ITU patients with significant corneal exposure or ulceration need follow-up at least weekly, more frequently in severe cases. Whilst ITU staff are traditionally skilled at protecting the eye with patches and lubricants, this system can break down so it is always worth checking this aspect of treatment as well.

PITFALLS

1. Missing anterior pathology whilst quickly rushing to review the fundus may miss something eminently treatable.
2. Inadequate follow-up or review with a different ophthalmologist on each occasion may make progress or treatment response assessment difficult, especially if the documentation is poor and the patient is ventilated and unable to give a subjective opinion. Try to follow the patient up yourself.
3. Good communication and documentation will be needed as multiple teams are often involved with ITU patients juggling their various problems.
4. ITU patients are complicated – don't be afraid to ask for senior input in the face of uncertainty.

FURTHER READING

Infectious Diseases Society of America (IDSA) 2016 Clinical Practice Guideline on Management of Candidiasis. *Clin Infect Dis.* 62(4); 2016 Feb 15.

25 When There Are Symptoms But it All Looks Totally Normal

Andrew Want

KEY POINTS

1. Was the examination truly normal or were subtle signs missed?
2. Consider causes that would warrant urgent imaging and management
3. Perform baseline examinations, measurements and investigations
4. Discuss with a senior ophthalmologist and arrange appropriate follow up

DIAGRAM OF ALGORITHM

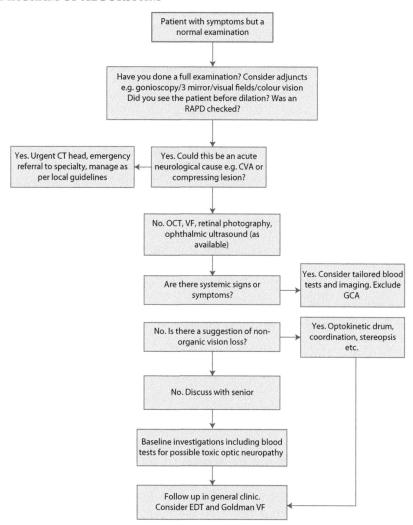

REFERRAL AND PRESENTATION

There will be times during your clinical practice in ophthalmology when a patient will complain of severe symptoms, and yet despite your hard work and with performing a detailed and thorough examination, you will not be able to find anything awry. This can be a very difficult and frustrating situation to manage. Despite deriving some reassurance from excluding serious conditions, the lack of a clear diagnosis can leave you feeling uneasy. There are a vast range of patient symptoms that may end up with a normal examination, such as flashing lights and floaters or headaches, all of which have been covered in previous chapters. Here we will focus on patients complaining of reduced vision or field loss. These symptoms may be monocular or binocular and may be acute or relatively long standing.

A detailed history is important with specific consideration of other general and systemic signs and symptoms. Details of any medications and exposure to other drugs or toxins at home or at work should also be sought out, especially if toxic optic neuropathy is a possible cause. Many genetic disorders may have minimal or no abnormal clinical signs in their early stages, and a detailed family history can give clues to a pattern of inheritance and possible diagnosis.

Non-organic vision loss (NOVL)/functional vision loss, defined as reduced visual acuity or loss of visual field that is not caused by any organic lesion, is also a possibility but is a diagnosis best reserved to last. It is more common in younger patients and females; however, it can occur in a wide variety of individuals. Thompson (1985) elegantly describes the spectrum of NOVL patients from the 'deliberate malingerer' who is intentionally trying to deceive for secondary gain, to the 'worried imposter', who invents symptoms but is genuinely concerned about a possible condition, the 'impressionable exaggerator' who tries to help the doctor by making their symptoms as easily identifiable as possible, and finally the 'impressionable innocent' who has convinced him- or herself that they have limited vision, often after a trivial injury. These patients can be challenging but some inquiry into their social history may help to reveal their motivations or an event that has triggered these complaints. Psychiatric disease is far from uniform in these patients, and many do not appear to have any psychiatric or personality disorder at all. It is also important to avoid the prejudice of assuming that a patient with mental health issues has NOVL, especially considering that several psychiatric medications have ophthalmic side effects with subtle signs, including ocular surface disease caused by anti-cholinergics, and pseudoparkinsonism from anti-dopaminergics causing a reduced blink rate.

DIFFERENTIAL DIAGNOSIS

The first consideration in this situation must be whether the examination was truly normal.

- Reflect on your assessment and consider any adjuncts to your examination such as using a gonioscope for eye pain or a three-mirror lens for hidden retinal breaks.
- Additional clinical tests and investigations you have available are outlined below.

After that, the priority in the emergency clinic setting is to determine if there is something that requires urgent investigation.

Intracranial pathology: The majority of these cases would include a central cause such as a stroke or space-occupying lesion. Rarely, pathologies such as an aneurysm or even a meningioma can present with subtle signs. Have a low threshold for requesting a CT head scan to aid diagnosis and consider an acute presentation a potential emergency. If only one eye is affected, this suggests a prechiasmal lesion, however, pathologies leading to a significant loss in vision would normally have a relative afferent pupillary defect (RAPD).

Giant cell arteritis: An atypical presentation of GCA should also be considered. Ensure you have asked about the associated symptoms and check for raised ESR and CRP if there are any doubts.

Retrobulbar optic neuritis: However, this is associated with definite symptoms and a typical history that should point the ophthalmologist in this direction despite the lack of clinical signs. Posterior scleritis may be entirely sign free but in practice a whole host of subtle changes, as well as additional testing with B-scan ultrasound, can give you vital clues.

Toxic optic neuropathy: Toxic optic neuropathy refers to visual impairment due to optic nerve damage caused by a toxin. It usually presents with gradual painless, symmetrical visual loss. Examination can be completely normal, especially in the early stages, or present with reduced optic nerve function and optic disc pallor with loss of retinal nerve fibre layer measurable on OCT. It can be caused by a wide variety of agents including medications, methanol, metals and tobacco. Nutritional deficiencies, especially vitamins such as thiamine (B1), riboflavin (B2), niacin (B3), pyridoxine (B6), cobalamin (B12) and folic acid, can also trigger it.

Others: There are many other rare conditions that present with minimal or no clinical signs especially in the early stages. These include Leber's hereditary optic neuropathy, Stagardt disease and acute zonal occult outer retinopathy. Generally these don't require any immediate management, and the role of the emergency ophthalmologist would be to exclude other treatable causes and collect accurate baseline information. Such diagnoses may require electrodiagnostic tests or genetic testing for confirmation, and management is often supportive and may involve genetic counselling with longer discussions with the patient and their family.

Refractive error: Previously undiagnosed amblyopia or refractive error should also be considered. If the patient has not had an eye examination in the past, then this may have gone unnoticed for many years. Be sure to ask if the patient ever had to wear a patch as a child or if they had any previous injuries or infections. Refer the patient to an optometrist for a formal assessment and correction as required. Remember you do not get an RAPD with poor vision due to amblyopia.

Functional vision loss: NOVL or functional vision loss includes a range of underlying conditions and disorders, with a complex mix of psychological and social elements. It is important to remember that NOVL is not a diagnosis of exclusion. There must be positive findings to demonstrate that the patient can see more than alleged. This may include the use of methods such as the optokinetic drum and Goldmann visual field as described below.

CLINICAL EXAMINATION

For this chapter, it will largely be assumed that a VA as well as a complete and accurate examination has already been performed. However, it is worth highlighting some specific parts of the clinical examination that can often be overlooked or missed, and can provide subtle but important clues to the diagnosis.

Pupillary reflexes: If the eye appears normal, the cause for a drop in vision may lie somewhere further down the optic pathway. A relative afferent pupillary defect

(RAPD) is an invaluable sign in a patient complaining of monocular vision loss. Perform the examination with the room lights dimmed and a strong light source such as the indirect headpiece. Ensure you check with the patient and staff whether they may have been dilated prior to your examination.

Colour vision: Colour vision is another useful part of the clinical assessment that can often be overlooked. If the patient's vision is too poor to use Ishihara pseudochromatic plates, a gross assessment using larger coloured objects and asking the patient to compare colour/red saturation in each eye may be helpful. This is one of the very few times the red hat pin you bought for visual field testing comes in useful.

Optic disc: Closely examine the optic discs, looking carefully for any subtle pallor, changes to the vasculature or any small disc haemorrhages. Make sure to examine both eyes in detail looking for any small differences between the two.

Visual fields (VF): Confrontational VF testing can be useful in an urgent care setting. While it may not be as reliable as an automated VF test, this is not always available. Pathology behind the optic chiasm will give a normal ocular examination with no RAPD, but may have a field defect. The patient may not have appreciated the true nature of the vision loss until testing and therefore may have presented as a generalised vision loss.

A VF, including those with a true defect, has a funnel shape, with the VF expanding moving further away from the eye. NOVL patients will often describe tunnel vision instead. Assess a patient's VF at 1 m using the standard technique. If a patient describes a constricted field, move back and repeat the test at 2 m. If the patient describes a similar size of field despite moving back, this is suggestive of NOVL (see Figure 25.1). Formal VF testing classically elicits cloverleaf patterns with Humphrey testing and spiraling with Goldmann.

Fogging: This is another method to try and demonstrate NOVL in patients with monocular vision loss. The patient is asked to read a vision chart with both eyes open. A trial frame is used with a neutral lens over the 'bad' eye, and a high power convex lens over the 'good' eye, obscuring the vision. Therefore, only the bad eye is being tested. By presenting the assessment as a binocular vision test, and by putting lenses over both eyes, the intention of the test is masked.

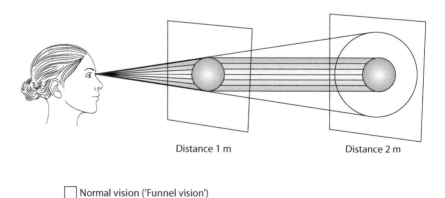

Distance 1 m   Distance 2 m

☐ Normal vision ('Funnel vision')

▤ Functional vision loss ('Tunnel vision')

Figure 25.1 Comparison of normal and NOVL/functional field loss.

Table 25.1: Relationship of Stereopsis for Visual Acuity

Stereopsis (Arc Second)	Visual Acuity
40	6/6
43	6/7.5
52	6/9
61	6/12
78	6/15
94	6/21
124	6/30
160	6/60

Source: Modified version of data from Levy N. S. E. B. Glick. *Am J Ophthalmol.* 78(4): Oct 1974; 722–724.

Stereopsis: Assessment of stereopsis can be particularly useful when the patient describes monocular vision loss. Stereopsis requires good vision in both eyes with good binocular fusion. Therefore if the patient can demonstrate good stereopsis, they must have good visual acuity. By describing the purpose of the test as being 'seeing how the two eyes work together', the true intention behind the test can be masked. During binocular tests it can be difficult to work out which eye is seeing and the patient may also try to close one eye during the test. The degree of stereopsis achieved can give some indication of the true visual acuity (see Table 25.1). Your orthoptist will hopefully assist you with this test.

Optokinetic drum: This is a simple device made up of a rotating drum with vertical lines on its sides. Looking at the rotating lines will elicit fast and slow phases of nystagmus in patients with at least 6/60 vision. This is an involuntary response to the moving stimulus and is therefore a more objective test (see Figure 25.2). The mirror test is a similar variation on the same principle. A mirror rotating on the vertical axis is positioned in front of the patient. The moving image on the mirror will produce a similar involuntary response.

Coordination tests: Simple tests of coordination and proprioception can also be useful to demonstrate NOVL. The patient can be asked to touch the tips of their

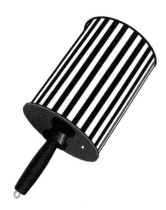

Figure 25.2 The optokinetic drum.

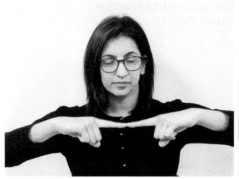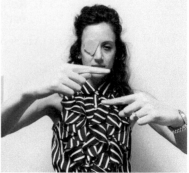

Figure 25.3 Coordination testing. The patient with NOVL (right) is unable to touch the tips of their index fingers.

index fingers together. This assesses proprioception and does not rely on vision. Therefore a patient with true vision loss will still be able to manage this without difficulty. A patient with NOVL will often claim to be unable to touch their fingers, as they believe the test is measuring their vision (see Figure 25.3). Similarly asking the patient to sign their own signature may cause similar outlandish aberrations in the belief that it is vision being tested. You can sign your own signature with your eyes closed. Try it.

Systemic examination: Loss of vision, especially with an acute presentation, may have a neurological cause. It is therefore important to look for any other focal neurological signs. Assess other cranial nerves, and perform an upper and lower limb neurological assessment. If a thrombotic cause is suspected, assess for atrial fibrillation and carotid bruits.

INVESTIGATIONS

OCT, retinal photography, automated visual field, ophthalmic ultrasound: Perform any immediate investigations you may have in the department such as formal visual field testing, OCT, retinal photography and ophthalmic ultrasound. These will help to give more clinical information that may help the diagnosis, but are also valuable baseline measurements that can be used for comparison at future follow-up appointments.

Blood tests: Always consider GCA in a patient with monocular vision loss, especially if there are other risk factors such as age or headache. Check ESR and CRP and if raised, manage as described in the earlier chapters. Urgent eGFR may be needed before giving contrast for a CT, as well as an urgent INR/coagulation profile if there is suspicion of a cerebral haemorrhage.

Toxic optic neuropathy can be caused by a wide variety of agents as well as some nutritional deficiencies. Blood tests should be taken to look for these abnormalities. Several medications, metals, methanol and tobacco can also cause toxic optic neuropathy so also include levels of any other specific agents as guided by the history and test availability (see Table 25.2).

CT head: If a central neurological cause is being considered, such as a stroke causing a new homonymous hemianopia, this should be treated as an emergency like any other stroke presentation. The medical team should be consulted and an urgent CT head should be performed. Consider orbital and sinus imaging depending on

Table 25.2: **Suggested Blood Tests**

General	Inflammatory Markers	Nutritional Deficiencies	Other
FBC	ESR	Folate	Specific drug/toxin
U&E	CRP	Iron profile	levels based on
LFT		Vit B1 (thiamine)	history
INR/clotting		Vit B2 (riboflavin)	
		Vit B6 (pyridoxine)	
		Vit B12 (cobalamin)	

history and examination findings. MRI can look at visual pathways in more detail for demyelination and inflammation.

Systemic investigations: Consider additional investigations such as chest x-ray and ECG as appropriate if there are any other systemic symptoms.

Electrodiagnostics and further investigations: During subsequent clinic follow up, it may be appropriate to request further imaging such as MRI, FFA or electrodiagnostic tests to further investigate the symptoms. However, these are specialist investigations and not usually ordered from the emergency clinic at the initial presentation. Goldmann visual field should also be considered in patients with suspected NOVL, as they will often show a characteristic spiral or star-pattern visual field as mentioned earlier.

DIAGNOSIS

When the examination is completely normal, it may not be possible to reach a final diagnosis until further investigations have been performed. Consider the differentials listed above and ensure you exclude those that would require urgent treatment. These will not usually be ordered from eye casualty; utilise the simple tests here to exclude sight threatening abnormality then refer to clinic and consider an orthoptist review.

MANAGEMENT

Review your examination and ensure it has been complete and that you have considered subtle signs. Never be afraid to ask a colleague to examine the patient as well if you have any concerns. For an acute history, the priority is to exclude an emergency condition. This will likely be a central neurological cause and should be immediately discussed with a senior ophthalmologist and appropriate specialties.

If an acute event such as a stroke or compressive lesion is considered unlikely, there may be very little to do in terms of immediate management. The goal should be to gather as much information to help guide further review. Discuss the case with a senior ophthalmologist and ensure any additional investigations have been requested based on the details of the presentation.

Reassure and be tactful with the patient (when NOVL is considered) and ensure all patients know to return if symptoms get worse.

FOLLOW UP

Arrange follow up in clinic at a time when the results of any pending investigations will be available, and chase the results of any important tests yourself. Depending on the onset of symptoms, a more urgent follow up in the coming days/weeks may be indicated to monitor the symptoms and assess if there is any further deterioration.

If a cause for the symptoms is found on radiological imaging, the patient will likely need referral to the appropriate specialty. Although the primary treatment and care will not be undertaken by the ophthalmology team, they may well require further monitoring for regular visual field tests and slit-lamp examination. The frequency and content of these appointments should be agreed upon with the other teams.

PITFALLS

1. Review your examination and consider whether it was truly normal. Think about whether you have seen the patient before dilating drops were given, and therefore could an important sign such as a subtle RAPD have been overlooked.
2. Never be afraid to ask a colleague or senior to examine the patient as well if you have any concerns.
3. Consider conditions such as a central neurological cause or an atypical presentation of GCA that would need urgent treatment.
4. Remember that non-organic vision loss is not a diagnosis of exclusion, but requires positive findings to demonstrate that the patient can see more than they are claiming.

FURTHER READING

Bruce, B. B., N. J. Newman. Functional visual loss. *Neurol Clinics*. 28(3): 2010; 789–802.

Kramer, K. K., F. G. La Piana, B. Appleton. Ocular malingering and hysteria: Diagnosis and management. *Survey Ophthal*. 24(2): 1979; 89–96.

Lessell, S. Nonorganic visual loss: What's in a name? *Am J Ophthalmol*. 151(4): 2011; 569–571.

Levy, N. S., E. B. Glick. Stereoscopic perception and Snellen visual acuity. *Am J Ophthal*. 78(4): 1974; 722–724.

Lim, S. A., R. M. Siatkowski, B. K. Farris. Functional visual loss in adults and children patient characteristics, management, and outcomes. *Ophthalmology*. 112(10): 2005; 1821–1828.

Miller, B. W. A review of practical tests for ocular malingering and hysteria. *Survey Ophthalmol*. 17(4): 1973; 241–246.

Thompson, H. S. Functional visual loss. *Am J Ophthal*, 100(1): 1985; 209–213.

26 Triage

Amy-lee Shirodkar

KEY POINTS

1. Always note down the patient's name, DOB, hospital/NHS number and contact phone number
2. Always take the referrer's name, job title and specialty
3. Identify the life/sight-threatening pathology first
4. Inform your eye casualty team of pending emergency cases to allow for the early preparation of necessary resources

DIAGRAM OF ALGORITHM

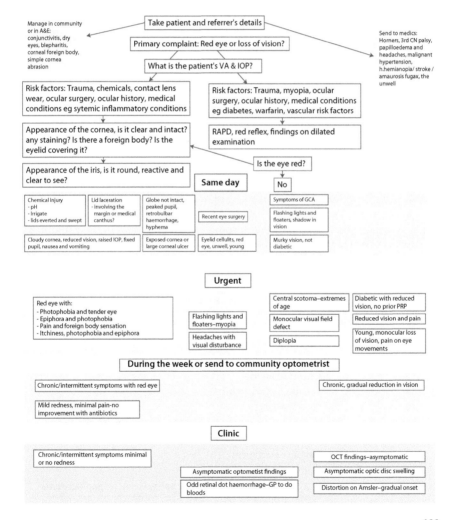

REFERRAL AND PRESENTATION

Triage is important in ophthalmology to help direct high risk pathology for urgent specialist care and low-risk pathology away from emergency ophthalmology services. It is a method of risk stratification, whereby the person triaging should obtain the necessary information from the referrer to decide how urgently the case needs to be seen, in what order and under what service. For example, an inexperienced junior doctor in a busy ED, nearing the end of their shift, is calling you about an adult patient with a swollen eyelid. It is up to you to decide in this case: What is the emergency? (1) Does the patient need an ophthalmology review? (2) When and where? (3) Is the optic nerve or eye compromised? (4) Any treatment required, what and how? (5) Does the patient need admitting, are they systemically unwell? So from the referral, eyelid swelling is not enough information alone to answer any of the above.

There are approximately 10 ocular emergencies that should be seen on the day as close to referral as possible due to their life or sight-threatening complications, see Tables 26.1 and 26.2. Those with a poor visual prognosis, if not treated in a timely fashion, will have permanent implications for the patient and medicolegal issues may arise if missed or mistreated. So always document the outcome of your triage decision.

Emergency ophthalmology services in the majority of cases are not the first port of call for patients with an eye problem. Most referrals come from GPs, local optometrists (accredited or not), A&E and other hospital specialties. Triage may be undertaken via telephone referrals, in house triage with the patient at walk-in services or scrutinisation of paper/digital referrals or a combination of all. Triage may be undertaken by you or another member of your urgent eye care team, but at some point the triage will be up to you, whether it be on the telephone whilst simultaneously undertaking a consultation for another patient or in the middle of the night, whilst on call.

Follow the algorithms in this book and the rest will come with experience as such to what specific questions to ask to rule out a penetrating injury versus a corneal abrasion, for example, and when to divert non-ocular conditions away, whilst reassuring the referrer. Ideally with time, you will be able to identify the potential diagnosis over the phone with minimal findings the inexperienced referrer offers; however, if faced with someone not confident in their findings or in situations where you want some more information, reassure, teach and explain

Table 26.1: A List of 'Red Flag' Ocular Emergencies that Need to be Seen on the Day of Referral

Ocular Emergencies

1	Endophthalmitis
2	Acute angle closure glaucoma
3	Chemical injuries
4	Penetrating eye injuries
5	GCA – AION
6	Severe ocular surface disease – Corneal melts/perforation
7	Corneal ulcers
8	Retinal detachment
9	Corneal exposure
10	Medical emergencies: third CN palsy, Horners, papilloedema

Table 26.2: A List of Urgent Ocular Conditions that Should be Seen as Soon as Possible

Urgent Ocular Conditions

1	Uveitis
2	Small corneal ulcers
3	Retinal tears
4	Non-nectrotizing scleritis
5	Macular haemorrhage – Wet AMD, Valsalva, traumatic

to them what to look for; they can always ring you back so you can make a better informed decision.

DIFFERENTIAL DIAGNOSIS

See Tables 26.1 and 26.2.

Urgent vs Non Urgent

In your mind, with the information given, you must formulate your differential diagnosis with the most serious pathology first. These include the duration of onset (rapid, sudden versus long, chronic and gradual), the degree of vision affected (snellen and RAPD), the IOP and associated risk factors – trauma, chemical contact, myopia (RD), ocular surgery and contact lens wear, for example. If the findings such as VA, or clinical signs rule out these top serious conditions then identify when and where the patient should be seen and whether the referrer can instigate any treatment in the meantime.

Emergency cases that you should see straight away, where visual prognosis is treatment time-dependent, include:

- Retrobulbar haemorrhage

- CRAO or suspect GCA with ocular symptoms

- Endophthalmitis

- Globe rupture/penetrating injuries

- Severe chemical injuries

- Angle closure glaucoma

- Orbital cellulitis

CLINICAL EXAMINATION

Telephone triage: Obtain enough information about the patient demographics, history, risk factors, optic nerve function and integrity of the eye from your referrer. Ask them what the visual acuity is, what the eye looks like, establishing corneal clarity, areas of staining, pupil shape and reaction. If your referrer can obtain photographic images, those will assist in your triage. Trained optometrists will be able to dilate and view the fundus so get them to describe their findings. Can someone check the IOP for you?

Patient triage: Gather information about the onset of symptoms. Acute? Have they waited a month to present? Can they be seen in a general clinic instead of in your urgent eye care service? Explain why their condition can wait for the duration specified, so the patient (and referrer) do not needlessly worry until then.

INVESTIGATIONS

After triaging the referral or patient complaint, give instructions about pre-consultation tests the patient can undergo before sitting in front of the casualty officer if it will affect the management of the case. Examples include BP, bloods for GCA, colour vision, RAPD, dilation, OCT and visual fields.

DIAGNOSIS

Essentially the diagnosis is made after clinical examination, but a lot can be assumed with the basic information and exposure to urgent eye care services through pattern recognition and experience. *Telephone triage:* With the history and basic examination findings you should be able to formulate a list of differentials in your head, if not be given the diagnosis by the referrer, for example, retinal detachment, dendritic HSK ulcer, or contact lens related ulcer. *Patient triage:* Again, you can formulate a differential on history taking or clearly observe the problem when speaking face-to-face with the patient. If you have triaged a referral, observe the outcome so you can manage such cases better in the future.

MANAGEMENT

Once you have gained enough information to formulate a differential diagnosis, decide whether you have an emergency, urgent or low risk condition before you. Those less urgent can be given medication in the interim by the referrer. For those more urgent, arrange where and when the patient should go for you to examine them, find out how long it will take and how they are going to get here. Remind patients not to drive if you think dilation may be indicated, and make sure the referrer gives the patient a referral letter to give you on arrival.

Arrange your eye casualty patients according to the most time-dependent. Then prioritise children, the vulnerable and in-patients. Manage your time well, especially whilst on call, spreading out patients so you take your breaks and consider how to fit in inpatient ward reviews.

Always inform your waiting patients on your progress, as they may feel hard done by when they see you calling patients in that arrived after them because you deemed them more urgent.

Request investigations before you see the patient where available to aid your consultation, such as OCT and visual fields.

Good communication will allow for the prioritisation of the correct patients, with appropriate work up and review by the appropriate member of the team. Continually communicate with your other urgent eye care colleagues to delegate tasks, ask for help or assist when called upon to ensure good team work and to ensure the that timely interventions and tests are performed.

In the rare occasion where you are faced with two equally time-dependent emergencies, ask for help or delegate tasks to ensure you are dealing with the most appropriate case.

FOLLOW UP

Certain ocular emergencies will require daily or twice daily review, or even admission.

For low risk conditions, explain and reassure the patient that their condition is not urgent and allocate them an appointment for the correct service in the most suitable time frame. Always ask the patient to chase up appointments if they haven't heard anything in the time frame you deem appropriate.

If in doubt, always ask for senior review or opinion, and consider bringing a patient in on a day when the sub-specialty team is available, where appropriate.

PITFALLS

1. Not taking a directed history including risk factors, e.g. are they a contact lens wearer.
2. Not taking the patient and referring party's details.
3. Not probing enough or asking the referrer to re-examine the patient for signs you need to rule out serious pathology.
4. Not reassuring the patient or referrer over the phone for those with likely low risk pathology.
5. Not sending patients through established pathways, e.g. wet AMD, asymptomatic optic disc swelling.
6. Accepting review of unwell patients that are better placed in a medical setting where out-patient ophthalmology departments are not.
7. Not having a triage structure and not sharing them with your referrers.

FURTHER READING

Denniston A., P. Murray. *Oxford handbook of Ophthalmology*, 3rd edition. Oxford University Press, 2014.

Jackson T. L., *Moorfields Manual of Ophthalmology*, Second edition, JP Medical Ltd, 2014.

27 Summary of Approach

Gwyn Samuel Williams

After the patient sits down and the history taking starts, tailor the questions so that your time is used most efficiently using the information given on the referral. If, for example, you suspect a corneal issue, concentrate on appropriate questions such as contact lens use and previous eye surgery; there is no need to ask questions about peripheral neurology that may be more appropriate for optic neuritis. Time is precious so make the most of every question you ask. Some casualty officers are excellent historians in that they ask every question imaginable though they then run so far behind that they incur the wrath of both patients and staff alike.

By the time you're ready to examine the patient, you should already be reasonably confident in what you expect to find. If the history, for example, is indicative of a retinal pathology then expect to find not much of anything on examination of the anterior segment and that pupil dilation will be required. Alternatively if the history appears to be related to trauma of some kind, then there will almost certainly be something to find superficially. Examination of the anterior segment should never be a fishing exercise undertaken because the history was nebulous and non-specific in order to find some guidance somewhere toward where the problem lies. No guidance will be found therein. As with the history, the examination must be tailored; there are many different tests and it is impossible to do everything as there is simply no time.

Once we reach the investigation stage, what needs to be done should be self-apparent even before the examination has come to an end. Do only what you need to do in eye casualty. Do not do anything extra. There is no time. Treat eye casualty as you would accident and emergency. Your role is to triage and make safe, not to correct every single problem in every single way for every single patient. Do not waste time on ordering tests that will not change management in the short term. A patient with a corneal ulcer will need scrapes undertaken immediately as you are about to start topical antibiotics, but a patient with a retinal vein occlusion is hardly likely to have an intravitreal injection in eye casualty for macular oedema. Management of retinal vein occlusion will entail recognition of the problem, assessment of severity with particular emphasis on intraocular pressure and presence or absence of neovascularisation as this may indicate that treatment is needed as a priority. Similarly, measure blood pressure and perform appropriate blood tests. Do not order fluorescein angiograms in eye casualty for anything other than suspected age-related macular degeneration. Do not order imaging unless there is a potentially life threatening pathology at play. Sometimes consultants when contacted will give casualty doctors a long list of tasks to complete; this is simply an example of getting a stressed, busy junior doctor to do tasks that would otherwise need to be completed in a specialty clinic. Do only what needs to be done.

Once the diagnosis is known and investigations, if relevant, ordered, the last step is to arrange for the patient to be either discharged or followed up appropriately in the hospital itself. Always remember to safety-net. Sometimes follow up is needed in eye casualty but for conditions that need specialist input the sooner they are discharged from the usually highly overstretched emergency system and into the right clinic the better it is for everyone. Resist the urge to bring everyone back ad nauseam with no plan and no idea!

Manage patient expectations, explain why they are experiencing the symptoms they are, when they should expect it to improve, and for those that aren't going to improve, tell them they won't go blind – reassure and reduce your patient's anxiety. Patient leaflets and an explanation of the treatment are always needed, but the emergency department is absolutely not the place for long chats and discussions. That said, reassuring a patient with trivial pathology that they aren't in fact going blind is an important function of eye casualty. Efficiency is key in running an effective emergency service. If you identify that a patient requires or is seeking a longer explanation or needs careful step-by-step instructions to improve treatment compliance, involve the eye clinic liaison officer or nursing staff so that you can be freed to see more patients.

We hope that you find this book useful in focusing attention toward what needs to be done. Do only what needs to be done. Focus from the beginning. Target examination and investigation. Eye casualty is daunting for most everyone but as gold is refined in the hottest fires, it is perhaps no coincidence that the best ophthalmologists have done more than their fair share of emergency work. Good luck!

28 The Moral Ophthalmologist

Gwyn Samuel Williams

Arrive early. While long delays might be considered par for the course when dealing with emergencies, do at least what you can to minimise problems for the patient, for the nursing staff, for your colleagues and ultimately for yourself. Patients are, as a rule, more distressed when they attend hospital as an emergency than when they attend routine appointments. They wonder if they are going blind, if they need surgery, if they need to arrange childcare, if they have their diabetic medication and if their relative who is out there parking the car will ever find them. What they don't like to see, therefore, is their doctor turning up late and then spending time chatting to the nursing staff, when all the while a roomful of waiting patients is staring on in quiet disbelief. Arrive early and don't chat to nursing staff or indeed anyone in a public place. If you wish to tell people how you found Rome or what you think of the latest mess the Tory party is up to, do this if you must behind a closed clinic room door or around the corner. Appearances are everything.

Know local guidelines and processes. Every hospital does things slightly differently, and it is imperative you know where the corneal scrape plates are kept, the laser room is, the codes to the drug cabinet and the way to order scans and book patients for emergency theatre. Expect to need this information at some point and knowing in advance is much better than trying to find out in the middle of a busy clinic. If you are allocated some time to get acquainted with a hospital, use it wisely. It is sadly not that infrequent that new doctors who are acting in a supernumerary capacity initially waste their time by seeing as few patients as possible and slinking away early as 'there are no patients booked for me'. This shows great disrespect to your colleagues in the clinic, and it is much better to act as a full member of the team from the outset. Otherwise a period of being supernumerary is utterly pointless.

Work fast and work smart. Time is important so try to be as in control of it as you can. Tailor your questions, your examination and your investigations. Do not waste time asking questions that do not alter what you do and do what you do need to do quickly. A detailed history is commendable but absolutely nobody will respect you for this if there is a still a gigantic number of patients waiting at the end of your shift. It is in fact quite immoral to insist on protecting yourself medicolegally as much as you can by writing copious notes and taking your time when patients and colleagues suffer because of it. Be concise and think of others.

Follow up your own patients. If you don't know what is going on, it is tempting to bring a patient back to someone else's clinic. Perhaps they can work out what is going on. Perhaps they can sort out what you can't. Similarly if you see a retinal tear, treat it yourself. Do not dump on others. If you do not know how to laser tears, learn. If you think a patient has giant cell arteritis investigate it yourself. It is absolutely not acceptable to bring back patients to another doctor's clinic and have the bare-faced cheek to write things such as 'consider GCA' in the notes, thereby protecting yourself and causing problems for others. If you think they should consider GCA then 'consider' it yourself. It may well be annoying having to wait for blood tests to come back, but it is much more work for someone else unfamiliar with the case to do it rather than you. Following up your own patients is the best way to learn because you are forced to know things yourself and take responsibility for your own actions. It is best for the patient too. There will always be doctors who take advantage of the system, but don't be one of them. Some people also like to decant responsibility for their own decisions on to a senior colleague by calling them up and 'discussing' the patient, so that they can then write this clearly in the notes. Discuss things with senior colleagues if you need genuine assistance with the decision-making process, but not to simply pass the buck.

Play fair. If there are multiple doctors in an eye casualty picking patients from a single pile of notes, as tempting as it may be, do not look through them and choose to see only what you want to see. If the next patient is a possible retinal detachment for example, and in your unit getting hold of VR is a complete nightmare, don't be tempted to take the rust ring underneath instead. You may get away with it once or twice but people are clever and they absolutely will work out that you are cherry picking patients and your reputation as a team player will be forever tarnished. We all know people who do this and we all talk about them; do not be that person. Similarly when the clinic comes to an end and there is one set of notes remaining, be the person to take it. There is honour in working hard, seeing the most patients, sorting out the most difficult problems and seeing the last patient. In some places in order to be able to leave earlier, sometimes there is a Mexican standoff over the last set of notes whereby everyone is 'just finishing off' something. Then finally when the last patient is taken in by a doctor, these tasks suddenly all come to an end and everyone else decamps for the canteen/home. If everyone looks out for everyone else then eye casualty is not so bad. It must also be remembered, however, that quantity is not always quality and some patients do take longer. Don't cut any corners but equally don't be that doctor whose work is of such 'quality' that they see so few patients relative to everyone else.

Don't avoid eye casualty. There seems to be a disproportionate amount of annual leave and sick leave that takes place during scheduled eye casualty clinic days compared to theatre days. Avoiding your duty causes delays to patient care and dumps quite massively on your friends and colleagues. People have to be pulled from theatre to cover and sometimes clinics and study leave sessions are cancelled. Do your duty. Work together for a happier eye clinic.

See all your patients. There are few things worse than arriving to an overbooked emergency clinic, but one of these is having to see your colleague's patients before even starting your own. Eye casualty is not like accident and emergency in most places. It is a booked clinic with slots. Admittedly sometimes particular patients take longer, but don't be that person who sees the end of their shift approach and then leaves remaining patients for someone else to see, finish your clinic like any other. Medicine is a vocation and not a job. Your duty is to your patients and not your paycheck. Finish your work and leave only when the patients are all seen; it denigrates the profession and the institution if you think your right to go home on time trumps your duty to see all your patients, or at least to have done everything in your power to do so.

Eye casualty at your hospital can be an example of communist utopia or capitalist hell. Working together helps everyone, and looking out only for yourself can have a very corrosive effect on your colleagues and the environment in which everyone works. It brings daily challenges interspersed with the routine. Whether it be trouble with daily gritty blepharitis, to the complex orbital swelling, or the care-free young contact lens wearer who sleeps in their daily lenses, the vulnerable abused child or the elderly lonely patient losing vision with bilateral wet AMD, the eye casualty is where we can positively affect the future thoughts, care and visual outcome for each of our patients. As a casualty officer, being part of the patient journey from the chaos and worry of potentially going blind whilst waiting in the waiting room to a state of reassurance from your explanation, or satisfyingly treating a patient's pain that they have struggled with for days, is what emergency eye care is all about. There is much joy as well in teaching juniors how to perform tasks and manage patients. Some staff are naturally more stressed than others and by sharing the load and spotting stressed out colleagues', burnout can be avoided, sickness prevented and the service nourished. The most precious resource in any eye department is the staff.

No service is perfect; where you see inefficiencies try to improve them, make them safer and easier to work in. Improve it for your colleagues and patients even if you are moving on in a few months. The tragedy of the commons is not infrequently encountered here, and we are only really able to control what we do as individuals, but by doing what we can and working for the common good we can make everyone's life easier. The colourful side of urgent eye care is what makes the sub-specialty so attractive. On behalf of all the authors of this book, good luck and work hard!

Index

A

AACG, *see* Acute angle closure glaucoma
AAPD, *see* Absolute afferent pupillary defects
Absolute afferent pupillary defects (AAPD), 148
Abusive head trauma (AHT), 136, 138; *see also* Non-accidental injury
AC, *see* Anterior chamber
Acanthamoeba keratitis, 33–34; *see also* Contact lens keratitis
Acute angle closure glaucoma (AACG), 2
Acute eye conditions, 29; *see also* Contact lens keratitis; Corneal ulcers
Acute retinal necrosis (ARN), 96, 98
Age-related macular degeneration (AMD), 88
AHT, *see* Abusive head trauma
ALTE, *see* Apparent life threatening event
AMD, *see* Age-related macular degeneration
American College of Rheumatology 1990 GCA classification criteria, 158
Anterior chamber (AC), 55; *see also* Sudden visual loss
    paracentesis, 63
Anterior segment ischaemia (ASI), 58
Anterior uveitis, 45; *see also* Photophobia
    granulomatous, 46
Apparent life threatening event (ALTE), 137
ARN, *see* Acute retinal necrosis
Arteriovenous malformation, 82; *see also* Suspicious retinal lesion
ASI, *see* Anterior segment ischaemia
Astrocytoma, 83; *see also* Suspicious retinal lesion

B

Bacterial ulcers, 32; *see also* Corneal ulcers
BAE, *see* Bleb-associated endophthalmitis
BETTS, *see* Birmingham Eye Trauma Terminology System
Birmingham Eye Trauma Terminology System (BETTS), 161
Bleb-associated endophthalmitis (BAE), 55–56
Blood pressure (BP), 104
Blurring, 87
BP, *see* Blood pressure
Brightness-scan (B-scan), 25, 55, 62, 84, *see* Ultrasonography
    IOFB, 163
    in obscured vitreous cavity, 73
    optic disc drusen, 61
    retina, 64

retinal haemorrhage, 70, 75
retinal tears and detachments, 70, 111
T-sign on ocular, 104
vitreous haemorrhage, 76
B-scan, *see* Brightness-scan
Bulging eyes, 115
    axial CT orbit of patient with TED, 119
    Clinical Activity Score, 118
    clinical examination, 117–118
    diagnosis, 119
    differential diagnosis, 116–117
    follow-up, 120
    investigations, 118
    management, 119–120
    management algorithm, 115
    pitfalls, 120
    referral and presentation, 116

C

Candida, 169
Capillary haemangiomas, 82; *see also* Suspicious retinal lesion
Carotid-cavernous fistula (CCF), 117
CAS, *see* Clinical Activity Score
Cavernous haemangiomas, 82; *see also* Suspicious retinal lesion
CCF, *see* Carotid-cavernous fistula
Cellulitis, 7; *see also* Eyelid swelling
    clinical examination, 9–10
    diagnosis, 11
    differential diagnosis, 8–9
    follow up, 13
    investigations, 10–11
    management, 11
    management algorithm, 7
    orbital, 12
    pitfall, 13
    pre-septal, 11
    referral and presentation, 8
Central retinal artery occlusion (CRAO), 60
Central retinal vein occlusion, 62; *see also* Sudden visual loss
CFD, *see* Congenital full disc
Choroidal; *see also* Suspicious retinal lesion
    melanoma, 80, 81
    naevus, 81
    neovascular membrane, 91
    osteomas, 82
Choroidal neovascularisation (CNV), 91
Clinical Activity Score (CAS), 118
CNV, *see* Choroidal neovascularisation
Computed tomography (CT), 118, 139

Congenital full disc (CFD), 147
Congenital hamartoma of retinal pigment epithelium, 83; *see also* Suspicious retinal lesion
Congenital hypertrophy, 83
Contact lens keratitis, 29; *see also* Corneal ulcers
  acanthamoeba keratitis, 33–34
  diagnosis, 32
  differential diagnosis, 30
  disciform keratitis, 33
  follow up, 36
  fungal keratitis, 34
  investigations, 31–32
  management, 34–35
  management algorithm, 29
  marginal keratitis, 30
  pitfalls, 36
  pseudomonas keratitis with corneal melt, 32
  referral and presentation, 30
  treatment, 35–36
  viral keratitis, 32–33
Coordination testing, 180
Cornea, 38; *see also* Corneal defect
  injury investigation test, 24
  issue management approach, 189–190
  layers of, 39
Corneal defect, 37, 38
  clinical examination, 39
  corneal abrasions, 37
  corneal foreign bodies, 37
  diagnosis, 40
  differential diagnosis, 38
  epithelial defect, 40
  follow up, 41–42
  investigations, 40
  management, 40–41, 189–190
  management algorithm, 37
  pitfalls, 42
  referral and presentation, 37–38
Corneal ulcers, 29; *see also* Contact lens keratitis
  bacterial, 32
  dendritic, 32
  diagnosis, 32
  differential diagnosis, 30
  follow up, 36
  investigations, 31–32
  management, 34–35
  management algorithm, 29
  pitfalls, 36
  referral and presentation, 30
  treatment, 35–36
CRAO, *see* Central retinal artery occlusion
C-reactive protein (CRP), 61
CRP, *see* C-reactive protein

Cystoid macular oedema (CMO), 90, 97
  causes of macular oedema, 92

D

Dacryocystography (DCG), 17
Dacryocystorhinostomy (DCR), 20
Dacryorhinocystotomy (DCR), 13
DCG, *see* Dacryocystography
DCR, *see* Dacryorhinocystotomy
Dendritic ulcer, 32; *see also* Corneal ulcers
Disciform keratitis, 33; *see also* Contact lens keratitis
Distorted vision, 87
  causes of choroidal neovascular membrane, 91
  causes of macular oedema, 92
  clinical examination, 89–91
  cystoid macular oedema, 90
  diagnosis, 91–92
  differential diagnosis, 88–89
  follow up, 93
  investigations, 91
  macular drusen, 90
  management, 92–93
  management algorithm, 87
  pitfalls, 93
  referral and presentation, 88
DON, *see* Dysthyroid optic neuropathy
Double vision, 123
  clinical examination, 124
  diagnosis, 126–127
  differential diagnosis, 124
  follow up, 127–128
  investigations, 126
  management, 127
  management algorithm, 123
  nine positions of gaze, 125
  pitfalls, 128
  referral and presentation, 123–124
Dysthyroid optic neuropathy (DON), 119

E

Eczema, 10
ED, *see* Epithelial defects
Endophthalmitis, 53; *see also* Red eye
  clinical examination, 54
  diagnosis, 56
  differential diagnosis, 54
  follow up, 57–58
  investigations, 55–56
  management, 56–57
  management algorithm, 53
  pitfalls, 58
  referral and presentation, 53
Epiphora, *see* Watery eyes

Epithelial defects (ED), 38, 40; *see also* Corneal defect
Erythrocyte sedimentation rate (ESR), 61, 91
ESR, *see* Erythrocyte sedimentation rate
Exophthalmometer, 116
Exophthalmos, *see* Proptosis
Eyelid swelling, 7
    bilateral, 8
    clinical examination, 9–10
    diagnosis, 11
    differential diagnosis, 8–9
    follow up, 13
    investigations, 10–11
    management, 11
    management algorithm, 7
    pitfall, 13
    racoon eyes, 9
    referral and presentation, 8
    typical S-shaped upper eyelid swelling, 9
    unilateral, 8
Eyelid trauma, 21–28

F

Facial investigations, 24–25
Facial trauma, *see* Ocular trauma
FB, *see* Foreign bodies
FBC, *see* Full blood count
FFA, *see* Fundus fluorescein angiography
Flashing lights and floaters, 67
    clinical examination, 69
    diagnosis, 71
    differential diagnosis, 68–69
    follow up, 72
    haemorrhagic PVD, 72
    investigations, 70
    management, 71–72
    management algorithm, 67
    pitfalls, 72
    posterior vitreous detachment with Weiss ring, 69
    referral and presentation, 68
    retinal detachment, 70
Floaters, *see* Flashing lights and floaters
Foreign bodies (FB), 30, 38
Fuchs heterochromic iridocyclitis, 48; *see also* Photophobia
Full blood count (FBC), 62
Functional vision loss, *see* Non-organic vision loss
Fundoscopy in fungal endogenous endophthalmitis, 169
Fundus fluorescein angiography (FFA), 61
Fungal endophthalmitis
    fundoscopy in endogenous, 169
    vitreous abscess, 171

Fungal keratitis, 34; *see also* Contact lens keratitis

G

GCA, *see* Giant cell arteritis
Giant cell arteritis (GCA), 126, 147, 153
    classification criteria, 158
    clinical examination, 156–157
    diagnosis, 158
    differential diagnosis, 155–156
    dilated, tortuose temporal blood vessel, 156
    follow up, 158
    investigations, 157
    management, 158, 159
    management algorithm, 154
    optic disc in anterior ischaemic optic neuropathy, 157
    pitfalls, 160
    referral and presentation, 155
    systemic and ocular manifestations of, 155

H

Haemangiomas, 82; *see also* Suspicious retinal lesion
Haematological malignancies, 81; *see also* Suspicious retinal lesion
Haemorrhages in vitreous, *see* Vitreous haemorrhages
Hamartoma of retinal pigment epithelium, 83; *see also* Suspicious retinal lesion
Headaches, 153
    classification criteria, 158
    clinical examination, 156–157
    diagnosis, 158
    differential diagnosis, 155–156
    follow up, 158
    giant cell arteritis, 155, 156
    investigations, 157
    management, 158, 159
    management algorithm, 154
    optic disc in anterior ischaemic optic neuropathy, 157
    pitfalls, 160
    referral and presentation, 155
HELLP syndrome (haemolysis, elevated liver enzymes, low platelets syndrome), 168
Hypertrophy, congenital, 83

I

ICP, *see* Intracranial pressure
Idiopathic intracranial hypertension (IIH), 64, 147
IIH, *see* Idiopathic intracranial hypertension

Intensive care unit (ITU), 168
Intensive care unit procedures, 167
    clinical examination, 170
    diagnosis, 170–172
    differential diagnosis, 169–170
    follow up, 173
    fundoscopy, 169
    management, 172–173
    management algorithm, 167
    pitfalls, 173
    Purtcher's retinopathy, 168
    referral and presentation, 168–169
    vitreous abscess, 171
Intracranial pressure (ICP), 145
Intraocular foreign body (IOFB), 22,
    75, 76, 162
    embedded in retina, 163
Intraocular lens (IOL), 89
Intraocular pressure (IOP), 4, 60, 63, 97
Intraretinal haemorrhages, 75
Intravenous (IV), 12
Intravenous methyl-prednisolone
    (IVMP), 119
IOFB, see Intraocular foreign body
IOL, see Intraocular lens
IOP, see Intraocular pressure
Iris neovascularisation, 74
Iritis, see Anterior uveitis
Irvine–Gass syndrome, 92
ITU, see Intensive care unit
IV, see Intravenous
IVMP, see Intravenous methyl-prednisolone

K

Keratic precipitates (KPs), 48, 49; see also
    Photophobia
Keratitis; see also Contact lens keratitis
KPs, see Keratic precipitates

L

Lateral canthotomy, 26
Leber's hereditary optic neuropathy
    (LHON), 147
Leukocoria, 129
    clinical examination, 132–133
    diagnosis, 133
    differential diagnosis, 131–132
    follow up, 133
    investigations, 133
    management, 133
    management algorithm, 129–130
    pitfalls, 134
    referral and presentation, 130
LHON, see Leber's hereditary optic
    neuropathy

M

Macular drusen, 90
Magnetic resonance imaging (MRI),
    118, 139
Marginal keratitis, 30; see also Contact lens
    keratitis
MECS, see Minor Eye Condition Service
Melanocytomas, 82; see also Suspicious retinal
    lesion
MG, see Myasthenia gravis
Minor Eye Condition Service (MECS), 46
MRI, see Magnetic resonance imaging
Myasthenia gravis (MG), 127

N

Naevus, 80; see also Suspicious retinal
    lesion
NAHI, see Non-accidental head injury
NAI, see Non-accidental injury
NAION, see Non-arteritic ischaemic optic
    neuropathy
Nerve fibre layer (NFL), 150
NFL, see Nerve fibre layer
Non-accidental head injury (NAHI), 136
Non-accidental injury (NAI), 135
    abusive head trauma, 138
    clinical examination, 137–142
    diagnosis, 142
    differential diagnosis, 136
    follow up, 143
    management, 142–143
    management algorithm, 135
    paediatric ophthalmology, 140–141
    pitfalls, 143
    RCOPHTH proforma, 138, 139
    referral and presentation, 135–136
    RetCam handpiece, 142
Non-arteritic ischaemic optic neuropathy
    (NAION), 155
Non-organic vision loss (NOVL), 176
    and normal field loss, 178
NOVL, see Non-organic vision loss

O

OCT, see Optical coherence tomography
Ocular; see also Sudden visual loss
    imaging, 62–63
    investigations, 24–25
Ocular conditions
    red flag emergencies, 184
    urgent, 185
Ocular trauma, 21
    clinical examination, 23–24
    diagnosis, 22–23

drugs for, 27
follow up, 26, 28
investigations, 24–25
lateral canthotomy, 26
management, 25
management algorithm, 21
peaked pupil, 23
pitfalls, 28
referral and presentation, 22
Siedel positive test, 24
Ocular trauma management, 161
BETTS, 164
clinical examination, 162–163
diagnosis, 164
differential diagnosis, 162
follow up, 165
intraocular foreign body in retina, 163
investigations, 163–164
management, 164–165
management algorithm, 161
peaked pupil after globe rupture, 163
pitfalls, 165–166
referral and presentation, 162
ONTT, see Optic neuritis treatment trial
Open globe injury, 161
Ophthalmologist, 191–193
Optical coherence tomography (OCT), 61, 111, 141
Optic disc drusen (ODD), 61, 147; see also Sudden visual loss
Optic disc swelling, 145
clinical examination, 148–150
diagnosis, 151
differential diagnosis, 147–148
follow up, 152
investigations, 150
management, 151–152
management algorithm, 145–146
optic nerve assessment, 148–149
pitfalls, 152
referral and presentation, 146
thickness map of optic disc, 151
Optic neuritis treatment trial (ONTT), 148
Optokinetic drum, 179
Orbital cellulitis, 12, 127; see also Cellulitis
Orbital trauma, 127

P

Paediatric ophthalmology, 140–141
Painful eyeball, 101
clinical examination, 102–104
diagnosis, 105
differential diagnosis, 102
follow up, 105–106
investigations, 104–105
management, 105

management algorithm, 101
pitfalls, 106
referral and presentation, 102
symptoms and pathology, 103
T-sign on ocular B-scan, 104
Pain in temple, see Headaches
Panretinal photocoagulation (PRP), 71
Papilloedema (PE), 145, 147
PE, see Papilloedema
PED, see Pigmented epithelial detachment
Periorbital trauma, 21–28
Peripheral ulcerative keratitis (PUK), 30
PHMB, see Polyhexamethylene biguanide
Photophobia, 45
clinical examination, 46–48
diagnosis, 49–50
differential diagnosis, 46
follow up, 50
Fuchs heterochromic iridocyclitis, 48
grading flare, 47
investigations, 48–49
keratic precipitate distribution, 48, 49
management, 50
management algorithm, 45
pitfalls, 51
referral and presentation, 46
severity grade, 48
Pigmented epithelial detachment (PED), 89
Polyhexamethylene biguanide (PHMB), 35
Posterior uveitis, 95
acute retinal necrosis, 98
clinical examination, 97
diagnosis, 99
differential diagnosis, 96–97
follow up, 100
inflamed areas of eye, 96
investigations, 98–99
management, 99–100
management algorithm, 95
pitfalls, 100
referral and presentation, 96
Posterior vitreous detachment (PVD), 68, 73, 74, 108; see also Flashing lights
haemorrhagic PVD, 72
with Weiss ring, 69
Proliferative vitreoretinopathy (PVR), 74, 108, 109
Proptosis, 116; see also Bulging eyes
PRP, see Panretinal photocoagulation
Pseudomonas keratitis with corneal melt, 32; see also Contact lens keratitis
PUK, see Peripheral ulcerative keratitis
Purtcher's retinopathy, 168
PVD, see Posterior vitreous detachment
PVR, see Proliferative vitreoretinopathy

R

Racemose haemangioma, *see* Arteriovenous malformation
RCOPHTH proforma, *see* Royal College of Ophthalmologists NAI Proforma
Red eye, 1; *see also* Endophthalmitis
  after cataract surgery and other operations, 53–58
  causes of, 3
  clinical examination, 2
  diagnosis, 5
  differential diagnosis, 2
  everting upper eyelid, 4
  follow up, 6
  investigations, 5
  management, 5
  management algorithm, 1
  pitfalls, 6
  referral and presentation, 2
  surface pathology of eye, 4
  triage of, 3
Red flag ocular emergencies, 184
Relative afferent pupillary defect (RAPD), 10, 60, 110, 148, 177
RetCam handpiece, 142
Retina haemorrhages, 73, 75, 135, 136, *see* Non-accidental injury; Vitreous haemorrhages
Retinal hamartomas, 83; *see also* Suspicious retinal lesion
Retinal nerve fibre layer (RNFL), 150
Retinal tears and detachments, 107
  causes of pathological floaters, 109–110
  clinical examination, 110–111
  diagnosis, 111
  differential diagnosis, 108
  follow up, 112
  investigations, 111
  management, 112
  management algorithm, 107
  peripheral retinal break, 111
  pitfalls, 113
  proliferative vitreoretinopathy, 109
  referral and presentation, 107–108
Retinal vasoproliferative tumours, 82; *see also* Suspicious retinal lesion
Retinoschisis, 108
RNFL, *see* Retinal nerve fibre layer
Royal College of Ophthalmologists NAI Proforma (RCOPHTH proforma), 138, 139

S

Sarcoidosis, 46
Scanning laser ophthalmoscopy (SLO), 141

SCH, *see* Subconjunctival haemorrhage
Secondary hyphaema, 22
Shaken baby syndrome (SBS), 135, 136; *see also* Non-accidental injury
Siedel positive test, 24
SLO, *see* Scanning laser ophthalmoscopy
SOL, *see* Space occupying lesion
Space occupying lesion (SOL), 145
Spontaneous venous pulsation (SVP), 150
SRF, *see* Subretinal fluid
Standard Uveitis Nomenclature (SUN), 47
Strabismus, 129
  clinical examination, 132–133
  diagnosis, 133
  differential diagnosis, 131–132
  follow up, 133
  investigations, 133
  management, 133
  management algorithm, 129–130
  pitfalls, 134
  referral and presentation, 130
Subconjunctival haemorrhage (SCH), 54
Subhyaloid haemorrhages, 75
Subretinal fluid (SRF), 84
Subretinal haemorrhages, 75
Sudden visual loss, 59
  anterior chamber paracentesis, 63
  central retinal vein occlusion, 62
  clinical examination, 60
  diagnosis, 63
  differential diagnosis, 60
  follow up, 64–65
  investigations, 60–62
  management, 63–64
  management algorithm, 59
  ocular imaging, 62–63
  optic disc drusen, 61
  pitfalls, 65
  referral and presentation, 59
SUN, *see* Standard Uveitis Nomenclature
Suspicious retinal lesion, 79
  arteriovenous malformation, 82
  astrocytoma, 83
  capillary haemangiomas, 82
  cavernous haemangiomas, 82
  choroidal melanoma, 80, 81
  choroidal naevus, 81
  choroidal osteomas, 82
  clinical examination, 83–84
  diagnosis, 84
  differential diagnosis, 80
  follow-up, 85
  haemangiomas, 82
  haematological malignancies, 81
  investigations, 84
  management, 85
  management algorithm, 79

melanocytomas, 82
naevus, 80
organisation of posterior pole tumours, 80
pitfalls, 85
referral and presentation, 79–80
retinal hamartomas, 83
retinal vasoproliferative tumours, 82
SVP, *see* Spontaneous venous pulsation
Symptoms without abnormalities, 175
blood tests, 181
clinical examination, 177–180
coordination testing, 180
diagnosis, 181
differential diagnosis, 176–177
follow up, 181–182
investigations, 180
management, 181
management algorithm, 175
normal and NOVL field loss, 178
optokinetic drum, 179
pitfalls, 182
referral and presentation, 176
stereopsis for visual acuity, 179

T

TAB, *see* Temporal artery biopsy
TASS, *see* Toxic Anterior Segment Syndrome
TED, *see* Thyroid eye disease
Temporal artery biopsy (TAB), 157
TFTs, *see* Thyroid function tests
Thyroid autoantibodies, 11
Thyroid eye disease (TED), 115, 127; *see also* Bulging eyes
Thyroid function tests (TFTs), 11
Thyrotropin receptor antibodies (TRAbs), 11
TIA, *see* Transient ischaemic attack
Toxic Anterior Segment Syndrome (TASS), 55
TRAbs, *see* Thyrotropin receptor antibodies
Transient ischaemic attack (TIA), 60, 69
Traumatic corneal injury investigation test, 24
Trauma to eyelids and periorbital region, 21–28
Triage, 183
algorithm, 183
clinical examination, 185
diagnosis, 186
differential diagnosis, 185
follow up, 186
investigations, 186
management, 186
pitfalls, 187
red flag ocular emergencies, 184
referral and presentation, 184–185
urgent conditions, 185
urgent vs. non urgent, 185

TS, *see* Tuberous sclerosis
Tuberous sclerosis (TS), 83

U

Ultrasonography, 61
Urgent ocular conditions, 185

V

VA, *see* Visual acuity
Vascular endothelial growth factor (VEGF), 64
VEGF, *see* Vascular endothelial growth factor
VF, *see* Visual field
Viral keratitis, 32–33; *see also* Contact lens keratitis
Visual acuity (VA), 60, 148
relationship of stereopsis for, 179
Visual field (VF), 149, 178
Vitreoretinal (VR), 63
Vitreous haemorrhages, 73, 75
clinical examination, 75
diagnosis, 76
differential diagnosis, 74–75
follow up, 76–77
investigations, 76
iris neovascularisation, 74
management, 76
management algorithm, 73
pitfalls, 77
referral and presentation, 74
Vitritis, 95
VKH syndrome, *see* Vogt–Koyanagi–Harada syndrome
Vogt–Koyanagi–Harada syndrome (VKH syndrome), 109
VR, *see* Vitreoretinal

W

Watery eyes, 15
clinical examination, 17
diagnosis, 18–19
differential diagnosis, 16
follow up, 20
investigations, 17–18
management, 19–20
management algorithm, 15
nasolacrimal drainage, 16
pitfalls, 20
preparing lower eyelid and punctum for syringing, 19
referral and presentation, 16
Wavy lines, 87
WECS, *see* Welsh Eye Care Scheme
Welsh Eye Care Scheme (WECS), 46, 88, 102

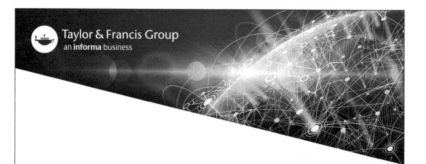

T - #0441 - 071024 - C218 - 234/156/9 - PB - 9780367110277 - Gloss Lamination